PROGRESS IN CLINICAL AND BIOLOGICAL RESEARCH

RECENT TITLES

Vol 288: **Immunity to Cancer. II,** Malcolm S. Mitchell, *Editor*

Vol 289: **Computer-Assisted Modeling of Receptor–Ligand Interactions: Theoretical Aspects and Applications to Drug Design,** Robert Rein, Amram Golombek, *Editors*

Vol 290: **Enzymology and Molecular Biology of Carbonyl Metabolism 2: Aldehyde Dehydrogenase, Alcohol Dehydrogenase, and Aldo-Keto Reductase,** Henry Weiner, T. Geoffrey Flynn, *Editors*

Vol 291: **QSAR: Quantitative Structure-Activity Relationships in Drug Design,** J.L. Fauchère, *Editor*

Vol 292: **Biological and Synthetic Membranes,** D. Allan Butterfield, *Editor*

Vol 293: **Advances in Cancer Control: Innovations and Research,** Paul N. Anderson, Paul F. Engstrom, Lee E. Mortenson, *Editors*

Vol 294: **Development of Preimplantation Embryos and Their Environment,** Koji Yoshinaga, Takahide Mori, *Editors*

Vol 295: **Cells and Tissues: A Three-Dimensional Approach by Modern Techniques in Microscopy,** Pietro M. Motta, *Editor*

Vol 296: **Developments in Ultrastructure of Reproduction,** Pietro M. Motta, *Editor*

Vol 297: **Biochemistry of the Acute Allergic Reactions: Fifth International Symposium,** Alfred I. Tauber, Bruce U. Wintroub, Arlene Stolper Simon, *Editors*

Vol 298: **Skin Carcinogenesis: Mechanisms and Human Relevance,** Thomas J. Slaga, Andre J.P. Klein-Szanto, R.K. Boutwell, Donald E. Stevenson, Hugh L. Spitzer, Bob D'Amato, *Editors*

Vol 299: **Perspectives in Shock Research: Metabolism, Immunology, Mediators, and Models,** John C. Passmore, *Editor,* Sherwood M. Reichard, David G. Reynolds, Daniel L. Traber, *Co-Editors*

Vol 300: **Alpha$_1$-Acid Glycoprotein: Genetics, Biochemistry, Physiological Functions, and Pharmacology,** Pierre Baumann, Chin B. Eap, Walter E. Müller, Jean-Paul Tillement, *Editors*

Vol 301: **Prostaglandins in Clinical Research: Cardiovascular System,** Karsten Schrör, Helmut Sinzinger, *Editors*

Vol 302: **Sperm Measures and Reproductive Success: Institute for Health Policy Analysis Forum on Science, Health, and Environmental Risk Assessment,** Edward J. Burger, Jr., Robert G. Tardiff, Anthony R. Scialli, Harold Zenick, *Editors*

Vol 303: **Therapeutic Progress in Urological Cancers,** Gerald P. Murphy, Saad Khoury, *Editors*

Vol 304: **The Maillard Reaction in Aging, Diabetes, and Nutrition,** John W. Baynes, Vincent M. Monnier, *Editors*

Vol 305: **Genetics of Kidney Disorders,** Christos S. Bartsocas, *Editor*

Vol 306: **Genetics of Neuromuscular Disorders,** Christos S. Bartsocas, *Editor*

Vol 307: **Recent Advances in Avian Immunology Research,** Balbir S. Bhogal, Guus Koch, *Editors*

Vol 308: **Second Vienna Shock Forum,** Günther Schlag, Heinz Redl, *Editors*

Vol 309: **Advances and Controversies in Thalassemia Therapy: Bone Marrow Transplantation and Other Approaches,** C. Dean Buckner, Robert Peter Gale, Guido Lucarelli, *Editors*

Vol 310: **EORTC Genitourinary Group Monograph 6: BCG in Superficial Bladder Cancer,** Frans M.J. Debruyne, Louis Denis, Ad P.M. van der Meijden, *Editors*

Vol 311: **Molecular and Cytogenetic Studies of Non-Disjunction,** Terry J. Hassold, Charles J. Epstein, *Editors*

Vol 312: **The Ocular Effects of Prostaglandins and Other Eicosanoids,** Laszlo Z. Bito, Johan Stjernschantz, *Editors*

Vol 313: **Malaria and the Red Cell: 2,** John W. Eaton, Steven R. Meshnick, George J. Brewer, *Editors*

Vol 314: **Inherited and Environmentally Induced Retinal Degenerations,** Matthew M. LaVail, Robert E. Anderson, Joe G. Hollyfield, *Editors*

Vol 315: **Muscle Energetics,** Richard J. Paul, Gijs Elzinga, Kazuhiro Yamada, *Editors*

Vol 316: **Hemoglobin Switching,** George Stamatoyannopoulos, Arthur W. Nienhuis, *Editors*. Published in two volumes: Part A: *Transcriptional Regulation*. Part B: *Cellular and Molecular Mechanisms*.

Vol 317: **Alzheimer's Disease and Related Disorders,** Khalid Iqbal, Henryk M. Wisniewski, Bengt Winblad, *Editors*

Vol 318: **Mechanisms of Chromosome Distribution and Aneuploidy,** Michael A. Resnick, Baldev K. Vig, *Editors*

Vol 319: **The Red Cell: Seventh Ann Arbor Conference,** George J. Brewer, *Editor*

Vol 320: **Menopause: Evaluation, Treatment, and Health Concerns,** Charles B. Hammond, Florence P. Haseltine, Isaac Schiff, *Editors*

Vol 321: **Fatty Acid Oxidation: Clinical, Biochemical, and Molecular Aspects,** Kay Tanaka, Paul M. Coates, *Editors*

Vol 322: **Molecular Endocrinology and Steroid Hormone Action,** Gordon H. Sato, James L. Stevens, *Editors*

Vol 323: **Current Concepts in Endometriosis,** Dev R. Chadha, Veasy C. Buttram, Jr., *Editors*

Vol 324: **Recent Advances in Hemophilia Care,** Carol K. Kasper, *Editor*

Vol 325: **Alcohol, Immunomodulation, and AIDS,** Daniela Seminara, Ronald Ross Watson, Albert Pawlowski, *Editors*

Vol 326: **Nutrition and Aging,** Derek M. Prinsley, Harold H. Sandstead, *Editors*

Vol 327: **Frontiers in Smooth Muscle Research,** Nicholas Sperelakis, Jackie D. Wood, *Editors*

Vol 328: **The International Narcotics Research Conference (INRC) '89,** Rémi Quirion, Khem Jhamandas, Christina Gianoulakis, *Editors*

Vol 329: **Multipoint Mapping and Linkage Based Upon Affected Pedigree Members: Genetic Analysis Workshop 6,** Robert C. Elston, M. Anne Spence, Susan E. Hodge, Jean W. MacCluer, *Editors*

Vol 330: **Verocytotoxin-Producing *Escherichia coli* Infections,** Martin Petric, Charles R. Smith, Clifford A. Lingwood, James L. Brunton, Mohamed A. Karmali, *Editors*

Vol 331: **Mouse Liver Carcinogenesis: Mechanisms and Species Comparisons,** Donald E. Stevenson, R. Michael McClain, James A. Popp, Thomas J. Slaga, Jerrold M. Ward, Henry C. Pitot, *Editors*

Vol 332: **Molecular and Cellular Regulation of Calcium and Phosphate Metabolism,** Meinrad Peterlik, Felix Bronner, *Editors*

Vol 333: **Bone Marrow Purging and Processing,** Samuel Gross, Adrian P. Gee, Diana A. Worthington-White, *Editors*

Vol 334: **Potassium Channels: Basic Function and Therapeutic Aspects,** Thomas J. Colatsky, *Editor*

Vol 335: **Evolution of Subterranean Mammals at the Organismal and Molecular Levels,** Eviatar Nevo, Osvaldo A. Reig, *Editors*

Vol 336: **Dynamic Interactions of Myelin Proteins,** George A. Hashim, Mario Moscarello, *Editors*

Vol 337: **Apheresis,** Gail Rock, *Editor*

Vol 338: **Hematopoietic Growth Factors in Transfusion Medicine,** Jerry Spivak, William Drohan, Douglas Dooley, *Editors*

Please contact publisher for information about previous titles in this series.

HEMATOPOIETIC GROWTH FACTORS IN TRANSFUSION MEDICINE

HEMATOPOIETIC GROWTH FACTORS IN TRANSFUSION MEDICINE

Proceedings of the XXth Annual Scientific Symposium of the American Red Cross, Held in Bethesda, Maryland, May 10–11, 1989

Editors

Jerry Spivak
Division of Hematology
Department of Medicine
Johns Hopkins Medical Institution
Baltimore, Maryland

William Drohan
Plasma Derivatives Laboratory
American Red Cross
Rockville, Maryland

Douglas Dooley
American Red Cross
Pacific Northwest Region
Portland, Oregon

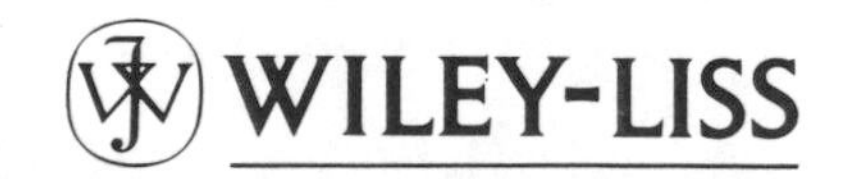

A JOHN WILEY & SONS, INC., PUBLICATION
NEW YORK • CHICHESTER • BRISBANE • TORONTO • SINGAPORE

nquiries to the Publisher
;t 11th Street, New York, NY 10003

Printed in United States of America

While the authors, editors, and publisher believe that drug selection and dosage and the specifications and usage of equipment and devices, as set forth in this book, are in accord with current recommendations and practice at the time of publication, they accept no legal responsibility for any errors or omissions, and make no warranty, express or implied, with respect to material contained herein. In view of ongoing research, equipment modifications, changes in governmental regulations and the constant flow of information relating to drug therapy, drug reactions and the use of equipment and devices, the reader is urged to review and evaluate the information provided in the package insert or instructions for each drug, piece of equipment or device for, among other things, any changes in the instructions or indications of dosage or usage and for added warnings and precautions.

The publication of this volume was facilitated by the authors and editors who submitted the text in a form suitable for direct reproduction without subsequent editing or proofreading by the publisher.

Library of Congress Cataloging-in-Publication Data

American Red Cross Scientific Symposium (20th : 1989 : Bethesda, Md.)
Hematopoietic growth factors in transfusion medicine : proceedings of the XXth Annual Scientific Symposium of the American Red Cross, held in Bethesda, Maryland, May 10-11, 1989 / editors, Jerry Spivak, William Drohan, Douglas Dooley.
p. cm. -- (Progress in clinical and biological research ; v. 338)
Includes bibliographical references.
ISBN 0-471-56761-2
1. Hematopoietic growth factors--Therapeutic use--Testing--Congresses. 2. Hematopoietic growth factors--Congresses. 3. Blood--Transfusion--Congresses. I. Spivak, Jerry L. II. Drohan, William. III. Dooley, Douglas. IV. Title. V. Series.
[DNLM: 1. Blood Transfusion--congresses. 2. Colony--Stimulating Factor--physiology--congresses. 3. Growth Substances--physiology--congresses. 4. Hematopoiesis--congresses. W1 PR668E v. 338 / WH 140 A512h 1989]
RM666.H25A44 1989
615'.39--dc20
DNLM/DLC
for Library of ... 9-21486
CIP

Contents

Contributors . . . . **ix**

Preface . . . . **xiii**

Biology of Hematopoiesis and Synergy Amongst Hematopoietic Growth Factors
Peter J. Quesenberry, Daniel Temeles, Marc Stewart, Ian McNiece, Helen McGrath, Donna Deacon, and Kotteazeth Srikumar **1**

Erythropoietin: Molecular and Cellular Biology
Eugene Goldwasser **19**

Human Granulocyte-Macrophage Colony-Stimulating Factor (GM-CSF): Regulation of Expression
Judith C. Gasson, John K. Fraser, and Stephen D. Nimer **27**

Macrophage Growth and Stimulating Factor, M-CSF
Peter Ralph and Adam Sampson-Johannes **43**

Interleukin-7: A New Hematopoietic Growth Factor
Anthony E. Namen, Douglas E. Williams, and Raymond G. Goodwin **65**

Cytokine Control of Human Megakaryocytopoiesis
Ronald Hoffman, Robert A. Briddell, John E. Straneva, John E. Brandt, Edward Bruno, Arnold Ganser, Norman Hudson, and Timothy Guscar **75**

Erythropoietin Therapy in Autologous Blood Donors
Lawrence T. Goodnough **105**

Erythropoietin Therapy in AIDS
David H. Henry **113**

The Use of Recombinant Human Granulocyte-Macrophage Colony-Stimulating Factor in Autologous Bone Marrow Transplantation
William P. Peters, Joanne Kurtzberg, Susan Atwater, Michael Borowitz, Murali Rao, Mark Currie, Colleen Gilbert, Elizabeth J. Shpall, Roy B. Jones, and Maureen Ross **121**

Cellular Interaction Regulating the Production of Colony-Stimulating Factors
James D. Griffin, George D. Demetri, Yuzuru Kanakura, Stephen A. Cannistra, and Timothy J. Ernst **129**

Effects of Recombinant Human Granulocyte-Macrophage Colony-Stimulating Factor as Treatment for Aplastic Anemia and Agranulocytosis
Richard E. Champlin, Stephen D. Nimer, Dagmar Oette, and David W. Golde **143**

Effects of Treatment of Myelodysplastic Syndromes With Recombinant Human Granulocyte Colony Stimulating Factor
Peter Greenberg, Robert Negrin, Arnon Nagler, Larry Souza, and Timothy Donlon **151**

Granulocyte Macrophage Colony Stimulating Factor (GM-CSF) in AIDS
David T. Scadden **163**

Index **177**

Contributors

Susan Atwater, Bone Marrow Transplant Program, Duke University Medical School, Durham, NC 27710 **[121]**

Michael Borowitz, Bone Marrow Transplant Program, Duke University Medical Center, Durham, NC 27710 **[121]**

John E. Brandt, Section of Hematology/Oncology, Department of Medicine, Indiana University School of Medicine, Indianapolis, IN 46202 **[75]**

Robert A. Briddell, Section of Hematology/Oncology, Department of Medicine, Indiana University School of Medicine, Indianapolis, IN 46202 **[75]**

Edward Bruno, Section of Hematology/Oncology, Department of Medicine, Indiana University School of Medicine, Indianapolis, IN 46202 **[75]**

Stephen A. Cannistra, Division of Tumor Immunology, Dana-Farber Cancer Institute, Boston, MA 02115 **[129]**

Richard E. Champlin, UCLA Center for Health Sciences and the Jonsson Comprehensive Cancer Center, Los Angeles, CA 90024 **[143]**

Mark Currie, Bone Marrow Transplant Program, Duke University Medical School, Durham, NC 27710 **[121]**

Donna Deacon, University of Virginia School of Medicine, Charlottesville, VA 22908 **[1]**

George D. Demetri, Division of Tumor Immunology, Dana-Farber Cancer Institute, Boston, MA 02115 **[129]**

Timothy Donlon, Stanford Medical Center, Stanford, CA 94305 **[151]**

Timothy J. Ernst, Division of Tumor Immunology, Dana-Farber Cancer Institute, Boston, MA 02115 **[129]**

John K. Fraser, Division of Hematology-Oncology, Department of Medicine, UCLA School of Medicine, Los Angeles, CA 90024 **[27]**

Arnold Ganser, Department of Hematology, University of Frankfurt, Frankfurt, Federal Republic of Germany **[75]**

Judith C. Gasson, Division of Hematology-Oncology, Department of Medicine, UCLA School of Medicine, Los Angeles, CA 90024 **[27]**

Colleen Gilbert, Bone Marrow Transplant Program, Duke University Medical Center, Durham, NC 27710 **[121]**

The numbers in brackets are the opening page numbers of the contributors' articles.

David W. Golde, UCLA Center for Health Sciences and the Johnsson Comprehensive Cancer Center, Los Angeles, CA 90024 **[143]**

Eugene Goldwasser, Department of Biochemistry and Molecular Biology, The University of Chicago, Chicago, IL 60637 **[19]**

Lawrence T. Goodnough, Department of Medicine and Pathology, Case Western Reserve University, Cleveland, OH 44106 **[105]**

Raymond G. Goodwin, Department of Molecular Biology, Immunex Corporation, Seattle, WA 98101 **[65]**

Peter Greenberg, Stanford Medical Center, Stanford, CA 94305 **[151]**

James D. Griffin, Division of Tumor Immunology, Dana-Farber Cancer Institute, Boston, MA 02115 **[129]**

Timothy Guscar, Section of Hematology/Oncology, Department of Medicine, Indiana University School of Medicine, Indianapolis, IN 46202 **[75]**

David H. Henry, Department of Medicine, University of Pennsylvania School of Medicine, Graduate Hospital, Philadelphia, PA 19146 **[113]**

Ronald Hoffman, Section of Hematology/Oncology, Department of Medicine, Indiana University School of Medicine, Indianapolis, IN 46202 **[75]**

Norman Hudson, Section of Hematology/Oncology, Department of Medicine, Indiana University School of Medicine, Indianapolis, IN 46202 **[75]**

Roy B. Jones, Bone Marrow Transplant Program, Duke University Medical School, Durham, NC 27710 **[121]**

Yuzuru Kanakura, Division of Tumor Immunology, Dana-Farber Cancer Institute, Boston, MA 02115 **[129]**

Joanne Kurtzberg, Bone Marrow Transplant Program, Duke University Medical School, Durham, NC 27710 **[121]**

Helen McGrath, University of Virginia School of Medicine, Charlottesville, VA 22908 **[1]**

Ian McNiece, University of Virginia School of Medicine, Charlottesville, VA 22908 **[1]**

Arnon Nagler, Stanford Medical Center, Stanford, CA 94305 **[151]**

Anthony E. Namen, Department of Experimental Hematology, Immunex Corporation, Seattle, WA 98101 **[65]**

Robert Negrin, Stanford Medical Center, Stanford, CA 94305 **[151]**

Stephen D. Nimer, Division of Hematology-Oncology, Department of Medicine, UCLA School of Medicine, Los Angeles, CA 90024 **[27, 143]**

Dagmar Oette, Sandoz Research Institute, East Hanover, NJ 07936 **[143]**

William P. Peters, Bone Marrow Transplant Program, Duke University Medical Center, Durham, NC 27710 **[121]**

Peter J. Quesenberry, University of Virginia School of Medicine, Charlottesville, VA 22908 **[1]**

Peter Ralph, Department of Cell Biology, Cetus Corporation, Emeryville, CA 94608 **[43]**

Murali Rao, Bone Marrow Transplant Program, Duke University Medical School, Durham, NC 27710 **[121]**

Maureen Ross, Bone Marrow Transport Program, Duke University Medical Center, Durham, NC 27710 **[121]**

Adam Sampson-Johannes, Department of Cell Biology, Cetus Corporation, Emeryville, CA 94608 **[43]**

David T. Scadden, New England Deaconess Hospital, Boston, MA 02215 **[163]**

Elizabeth J. Shpall, Bone Marrow Transplant Program, Duke University Medical School, Durham, NC 27710 **[121]**

Larry Souza, AMGen, Thousand Oaks, CA 91320 **[151]**

Kotteazeth Srikumar, University of Virginia School of Medicine, Charlottesville, VA 22908 **[1]**

Marc Stewart, University of Virginia School of Medicine, Charlottesville, VA 22908 **[1]**

John E. Straneva, Section of Hematology/Oncology, Department of Medicine, Indiana University School of Medicine, Indianapolis, IN 46202 **[75]**

Daniel Temeles, University of Virginia School of Medicine, Charlottesville, VA 22908 **[1]**

Douglas E. Williams, Department of Experimental Hematology, Immunex Corporation, Seattle, WA 98101 **[65]**

Preface

The purification and cloning of the hematopoietic growth factors erythropoietin, GM-CSF, G-CSF, M-CSF, and IL-3 have opened up new therapeutic vistas in hematology and, by extension, in medicine in general. For the first time, physicians have the opportunity to manipulate bone marrow function in both a positive and physiologic fashion and also with certain of these growth factors, to augment the functional activity of circulating leukocytes. Although the basic paradigm for the use of the recombinant hematopoietic growth factors has been to enhance hematopoietic cell proliferation in conditions where it is deficient, it is becoming apparent that these growth factors may be useful even when marrow function is normal but when increased demands on it are anticipated, such as in the case of autologous blood donors.

A paradox of the scientific achievements which brought the hematopoietic growth factors so rapidly into the clinical arena is that most clinicians are unfamiliar with them, since until recently these growth factors had been largely relegated to the domain of the experimental hematologist.

The goal of the XXth Annual Scientific Symposium of the American Red Cross was, therefore, to rectify this situation and, in particular, to explore the role of the hematopoietic growth factors in transfusion medicine. The need to conserve the nation's blood supply and to provide safe alternatives to blood transfusion has never been greater considering the anticipated increase in transfusion needs coupled with the well-documented infectious and immunologic hazards associated with the use of blood products.

To this end, a committee consisting of P.J. Quesenberry (University of Virginia), A.W. Nienhuis (National Institutes of Health), J.D. Griffin (Harvard University), W. Drohan and D. Dooley (American Red Cross), and J.L. Spivak (Johns Hopkins University) was organized to develop a symposium entitled **Hematopoietic Growth Factors in Transfusion Medicine**. The result was a highly successful scientific program which explored both the molecular aspects and clinical applications of not only the major hematopoietic growth factors but also the newer interleukins. In this volume, the manuscripts developed from the symposium presentations have been gathered together to provide a reference source for individuals wishing to expand their knowledge in this dynamic area.

Jerry L. Spivak

Hematopoietic Growth Factors
in Transfusion Medicine, pages 1–18

BIOLOGY OF HEMATOPOIESIS AND SYNERGY AMONGST HEMATOPOIETIC GROWTH FACTORS

Peter J. Quesenberry, Daniel Temeles,
Marc Stewart, Ian McNiece, Helen McGrath,
Donna Deacon, and Kotteazeth Srikumar
University of Virginia School of Medicine,
Charlottesville, Virginia 22908

INTRODUCTION

The colony stimulating factors and interleukins were initially defined as regulators for myeloid and lymphoid cells, respectively. With the purification and genetic cloning of these factors large amounts have become available for in-vitro and in-vivo testing and in several instances for clinical trials. It is now clear that these growth factors have a broad range of actions frequently overlapping and effecting multiple lineages. The colony stimulating factors, including granulocyte colony stimulating factor (G-CSF) (Nicola et al 1983; Nicola et al, 1985), granulocyte-macrophage CSF (GM-CSF) (Burgess et al, 1977; Gasson et al, 1984), colony stimulating factor-1 (CSF-1) (Waheed & Shadduck, 1979; Stanley & Guilbert, 1981; Stanley & Heard, 1977), and multi-CSF or interleukin-3 (IL-3) (Ihle et al, 1983a; Ihle et al, 1982; Yokota et al, 1984), were initially defined on relatively restricted myeloid lineages by their effects in stimulating colonies of these different lineages. For instance, G-CSF was defined as a factor which stimulated granulocyte colonies and could induce differentiation of certain murine myelocytic leukemia cells. GM-CSF was defined as an activity inducing granulocyte-macrophage colonies, CSF-1 an an activity inducing macrophage colonies, and IL-3 as an activity inducing multilineage colony formation including granulocyte-macrophage, megakaryocyte, eosinophil, basophil, and in the presence of erythropoietin, erythroid. With a fuller study of these activities it is clear that they all have certain aspects of multilineage action with the possible exception of CSF-1. G-CSF has clear actions as a pre-B inducer (Quesenberry, 1988) and acts on early myeloid cells (Ikebuchi et al, 1988) and on megakaryocytic lineages (McNiece et al, 1988a). GM-CSF acts across the spectrum of myeloid cells, is a direct megakaryocyte stimulator (Robinson et al, 1987; Quesenberry et al, 1985), a burst promoting activity for erythroid colony formation (March et al, 1985; Morgan et al, 1976), and also appears to have prominent effects on lymphoid pathways. Conversely, the interleukins (minus IL-3) were initially defined largely on T lymphocyte or B lymphocyte pathways, IL-1 having effects on both pathways and being a general modulator of growth factor production (Dinarello, 1984; March et al, 1985), IL-2 being a T cell stimulator (Morgan et al, 1976; Clark et al, 1984), and IL-4 through IL-7 being defined in various aspects of B lymphocyte proliferation and differentiation (Noma et al, 1986; Lee et al, 1986; Kinashi et al, 1986; Hirano et al, 1986; Tanabe et al, 1988; Hirano et al, 1985; Haegeman et al, 1986; Zilberstein et al, 1986; May et al, 1986; Van Damme et al, 1987; Namen et al, 1988a; Namen et al, 1988b; Sanderson et al, 1985). As with the colony stimulating factors, the interleukins with further study have been found to have a wide range of actions and to effect both lymphoid and myeloid pathways. A few examples include IL-6, initially defined as a B cell factor and now found to have potent activity on early myeloid stem cells, megakaryocytes and granulocyte-macrophage colony formation (Wong et al, 1988; Ikebuchi et al, 1987; Chiu et al, 1988; McGrath et al, 1989; Kawana et al, 1988). IL-5, another B cell factor, is perhaps the most prominent eosinophil colony stimulating activity (Schimpl & Wecker, 1972; Takatsu et al, 1980; Swain & Dutton, 1982; Campbell et al, 1987; Clutterbuck & Sanderson, 1988; Sanderson, 1988), IL-4, another B cell factor, clearly has prominent synergistic effects on various myeloid pathways (Lee et al, 1986; Broxmeyer et al, 1988; Peschel et al, 1987; Rennick et al, 1987) while IL-7, a recently defined pre-B cell stimulator (Namen et al, 1988a), now appears to have both T cell activity and activity in vivo in stimulating platelets in irradiated mice (Namen, 1989). These are a few observations underscoring the general phenomena of cross-lineage stimulation. Another important evolving theme is that of additive or synergistic actions of these various growth factors. A general rule has been that combinations of growth factors either give additive or synergistic effects in multiple assays on multiple different lineages. It is unusual not to see this type of synergistic or additive interaction between a variety of growth factors. Examples of this include in the erythroid pathway, the interaction of erythropoietin with IL-3, IL-4, GM-CSF and probably G-CSF to stimulate large erythroid colonies termed burst-forming units (Metcalf et al, 1986; Sieff et al, 1985; Peschel et al, 1987; Prystowsky et al, 1983) and the interaction of CSF-1 with G-CSF, GM-CSF, IL-3, and IL-1 to stimulate high proliferative potential colony forming cells (McNiece et al, 1982; Caracciolo et al, 1987; McNiece et al, 1988b; McNiece et al, 1988c; Stanley & Jubinsky, 1984; Jubinsky & Stanley, 1985; Mochizuki et al, 1987).

Another general feature of the action of these growth factors is that while defined usually at one phase of the differentiation sequence they appear to act in general throughout a differentiation cascade. Examples are GM-CSF and G-CSF which have actions on relatively early stem/progenitor cells but which also have major actions on multiple functions of granulocytes and monocytes in their pathways (Fleischmann et al, 1986; Metcalf et al, 1986; Vadas et al, 1983; Handman & Burgess, 1979; Aranout et al, 1986; Weisbart et al, 1985; Dispersio et al, 1987; Begley et al, 1986; Stanley & Burgess, 1983; Silberstein et al, 1986; Avalos et al, 1987; Wang et al, 1988; Vades et al, 1983). Similarly, CSF-1 acts at the progenitor/stem cell level and also is a major activator of mature macrophages (Wing et al, 1982; Wing et al, 1985; Ziboh et al, 1982; Hamilton et al, 1986; Lin & Gordon, 1979; Karbassi et al, 1989). Another general rule is that these growth factors appear to effect the neoplastic counterpart of their target cells with predominantly proliferative stimulation (Vallenga et al, 1987; Miyauchi et al, 1987; Ganser et al, 1989). This particularly important when considering the use of these factors in various clinical situations.

The stem cells and target cells of these factors have been most extensively worked out for the myeloid pathways and less so for the lymphoid pathways. However, conventional dogma suggesting that stem cells give rise to progenitor cells which give rise to restricted lineages may be replaced by a concept of definition of the progenitor/stem cells by their growth factor responsiveness. Figure 1 presents an overview of hemopoiesis which is clearly still in evolution showing points at which growth factors act and cells on which they act.

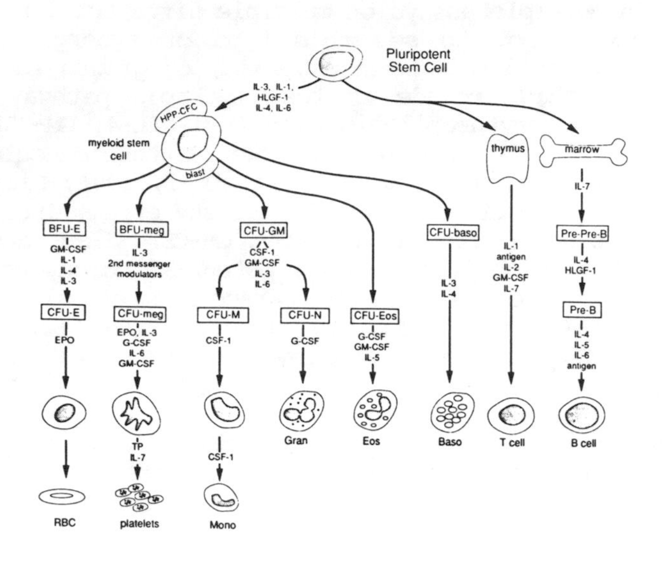

FIGURE 1. MODEL OF HEMOPOIESIS

An important consideration in evaluating the action of growth factors in either in-vitro or in-vivo settings is their potential effect on a variety of accessory cells. A large number of cells have now been established as capable of producing a wide variety of growth factors. The growth factors may either be detected by bioassay or alternatively by Northern blot analysis of mRNA. In some instances baseline production is established whereas in others various inducers have to be present in order to detect growth factor production. These inducers include IL-1, tumor necrosis factor, interferon, lectins, endotoxin and various other growth factors. This has led to the concept of constitutive versus induced production although given the sensitivity of the mRNA assays it is not clear whether most of these cells produce low levels of growth factor simply below the sensitivity of the methods used to detect growth factor bioactivity or mRNA levels. In any case, endothelial cells, fibroblasts, vascular smooth muscle, B cells, T cells, monocytes and a number of variants of these cell types have now been shown to produce multiple growth factors frequently including GM-CSF, G-CSF and CSF-1 (Zucali et al, 1986; Koeffler et al, 1987; Ramaldi et al, 1987; Horiguchi et al, 1987; Oster et al, 1987; Metcalf & Nicola, 1985; Bagby et al, 1986; Munker et al, 1986; Broudy et al, 1986; Kaushansky et al, 1987; Quesenberry & Gimbrone, 1980; Quesenberry & Gimbrone, 1983; Ihle et al, 1983b; Clark & Kamen, 1987; Gualtieri et al, 1984; Alberico et al, 1987; McGrath et al, 1987; Quesenberry & Levitt, 1979; Golde & Cline, 1972; Chervenick & LoBuglio, 1972; Moore & Williams, 1972; Parker & Metcalf, 1974; Cline & Golde, 1974; Song & Quesenberry, 1984; Quesenberry et al, 1987; Lovhaug et al, 1986; Bagby et al, 1983; Knudtzon & Mortensen, 1975; Guez & Sachs, 1973; Austin et al, 1971; Bickel et al, 1987; Quesenberry et al, 1981; Chodakewitz et al, 1988; Lee et al, 1988). IL-3 seems to be an exception in that it appears to be produced only by T lymphocytes (Ihle et al, 1983a; Clark & Kamen, 1987; Yang et al, 1986). Thus there is a great capacity for factor production by any cell population and observed effects might either be direct or via induction of these various growth factors. Evidence has evolved for the ability of a number of growth factors including GM-CSF, IL-3, IL-1, IL-6 and others to induce other growth factors or even to induce themselves in an autocrine-type style. This system gives the potential for tremendous modulation and redundancy in growth factor action. Thus it is important to emphasize that even at the single cell level, usually not obtained in most studies, actions of growth factors may in fact be mediated by production of other growth factors. Stromal marrow cells are also a very potent source of many different growth factors.

A general model of hemopoiesis can include two different settings for growth factor control of marrow cell production as exemplified by the granulocyte-monocyte system and the response to infection or endotoxin injection. Acute emergency situations such as might be represented by endotoxin injection or bacterial infection would appear to have the capacity to generate high levels of circulating growth factor produced by a variety of sentinel cells exposed to these challenges. These growth factors, probably including G-CSF, CSF-1 and IL-6, then have the capacity to both activate local cells and to stimulate the production of marrow cells. They also have the capacity to induce bone marrow stromal cell factor production to further augment the response. However, a good deal of data points to the importance of local bone marrow stromal cell factor production in the regulation of hemopoiesis. Observations of the growth of primitive stem cells directly on stromal cells and of the importance of stromal cells to ongoing hemopoiesis in long term liquid culture are consistent with earlier in vivo studies on the importance of the microenvironment (Friedenstein et al, 1970; Dexter et al, 1977; McGrath et al, 1987; Testa & Dexter, 1977; Williams et al, 1978; Williams et al, 1977; Greenberger, 1978; Doukas et al, 1985). Bone marrow stromal cells and stromal cell lines have been rich sources of multiple growth factors and appear capable of producing a number of different growth factors. These type of data suggest that an important mode of regulation may be the local presentation of multiple different growth factors possibly bound to core proteins to bone marrow stem cells. Data by Gordon and colleagues (Gordon et al, 1987) have suggested that proteoglycans may bind and present growth factors to stem cells and in a similar fashion membrane proteins or extracellular matrix proteins may bind a number of growth factors at very low concentration and present these to stem cells. This seems likely to be an important mode of stem cell regulation, the modulation of this system then being determined possibly by the ratios of growth factors, the absolute amounts or the actual configuration in which they are presented. Pulse high levels of peripheral circulating growth factors may then impact on such a baseline system to further define the final pathway of differentiation. The conventional model of sequential growth factor action is contrasted with this concept in Figure 2. A consideration of these models in the context of recent clinical trials might suggest that the actions of growth factors in clinical trials resembles the emergent type model with very high levels overriding normal control mechanisms. Thus the administration of G-CSF or GM-CSF probably represents the type of stimulus given when a mammal is exposed to a dangerous foreign stimulus. Thus it seems unlikely that administration of these factors mimics normal regulatory mechanisms although the end result may still be beneficial. Another important consideration with regard to the use of these growth factors clinically is the above noted action of these growth factors on neoplastic counterparts of their target cells and the possible wider action on other neoplasms. It is also important to keep in mind their prominent action on activating mature end cells. This could both be a major positive with regard to clearing of infection but also could activate inflammatory loci and lead to toxic

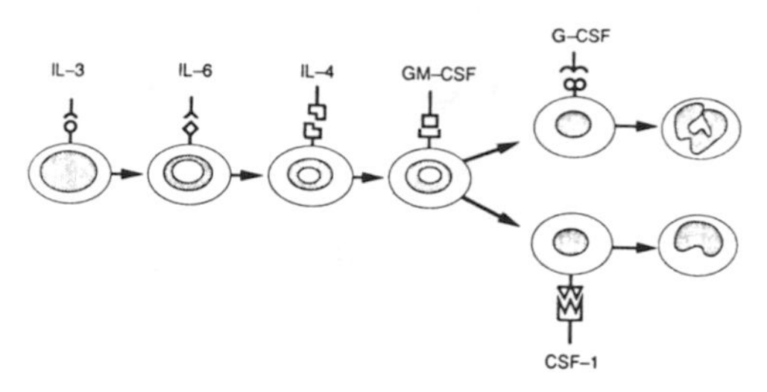

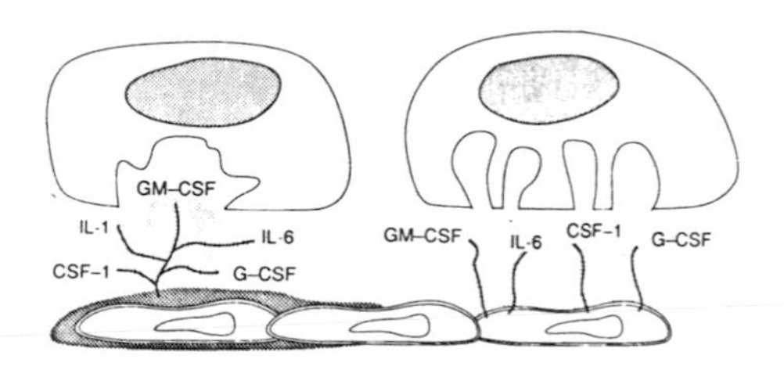

FIGURE 2. MODEL OF GROWTH FACTOR ACTION.

side effects. We can look forward to the introduction of combinations of growth factors into clinical trial, of new growth factors and the use of growth factors to synchronize neoplastic cells for cell cycle specific killing.

REFERENCES

Alberico T, Ihle JN, Quesenberry P (1987) Stromal growth factor production in irradiated lectin exposed long term murine bone marrow cultures. Blood 69:1120-1127.

Aranout MA, Wang EA, Clark SC, Sieff CA (1986) Human recombinant granulocyte-macrophage colony stimulating factor increases cell-to-cell adhesion and surface expression of adhesion-promoting surface glycoproteins on mature granulocytes. J Clin Invest 78:597-601.

Austin PE, McCulloch EA, Till JE (1971) Characterization of the factor in L-cell conditioned medium capable of stimulating colony formation by mouse marrow cells in culture. J Cell Physiol 77:121-134.

Avalos BR, Hedzat C, Baldwin GC et al (1987) Biological activities of human G-CSF and characterization of the human G-CSF receptor. Blood 70:165a (abstract).
Bagby GC, McCall Em, Layman DL (1983) Regulation of colony stimulating activity production: Interactions of fibroblasts, mononuclear phagocytes and lactoferrin. J Clin Invest 71:340-344.
Bagby GC, Dinarello CA, Wallace P, Wagner C, Hefeneider S, McCall E (1986) Interleukin-1 stimulates granulocyte-macrophage colony stimulating activity release by vascular endothelial cells. J Clin Invest 78:1316-1323.
Begley CG, Lopez AF, Nicola NA, Warren DJ, Vadas MA, Sanderson CJ, Metcalf D (1986) Purified colony stimulating factors enhance the survival of human neutrophils and eosinophils in vitro: A rapid and sensitive microassay for colony-stimulating factors. Blood 68:162-166.
Bickel M, Amstad P, Tsuda H, Sulis C, Asofsky R, Mergenhagen SE, Pluznik DH (1987) Induction of granulocyte macrophage colony stimulating factor by lipopolysaccharide and anti-immunoglobulin M-stimulated murine B cell lines. J Immunol 139:2984-2988.
Broudy V, Kaushansky K, Segal G et al (1986) Tumor necrosis factor type a stimulates human endothelial cells to produce granulocyte-macrophage colony stimulating factor. Proc Natl Acad Sci USA 83:467.
Broxmeyer HE, Lu L, Cooper S, Tushinski R, Mochizuki D, Rubin BY, Gillis S, Williams DE (1988) Synergistic effects of purified recombinant human and murine B cell growth factor-1/Interleukin-4 on colony formation in vitro by hematopoietic progenitor cells. J Immunol 141:3852-3856.
Burgess AW, Camakaris J, Metcalf D (1977) Purification and properties of colony stimulating factor from mouse lung-conditioned medium. J Biol Chem 252:1998-2003.
Campbell HD, Tucker WQJ, Hort Y, Martinson ME, Mayo G, Clutterbuck EJ, Sanderson CJ, Young IG (1987) Molecular cloning and expression of the gene encoding human eosinophil differentiation factor (interleukin-5). Proc Natl Acad Sci USA 84:6629.
Caracciolo D, Shirsat N, Wong GG, Lange B, Clark S, Rovera G (1987) Recombinant human macrophage colony stimulating factor (M-CSF) requires subliminal concentrations of granulocyte macrophage (GM-CSF) for optimal stimulation of human macrophage colony formation in vitro. J Exp Med 166:1851-1860.

Chervenick PA, LoBuglio AF (1972) Human blood monocytes: Stimulators of granulocyte and mononuclear colony formation in vitro. Science 178:164-166.

Chiu CP, Moulds C, Coffman RL, Rennick D, Lee F (1988) Multiple biological activities are expressed by a mouse interleukin-6 cDNA clone isolated from bone marrow stromal cells. Proc Natl Acad Sci USA 85:7099-7103.

Chodakewitz JA, Kupper TS, Coleman DL (1988) Keratinocyte-derived granulocyte/macrophage colony stimulating factor induces DNA synthesis by peritoneal macorphages. J Immunol 140:832-836.

Clark SC, Arya SK, Wong-Staal F, Matsumoto-Kobayashi M, Kay RM, Kaufman RJ, Brown EL, Shoemaker C, Copeland T, Oroszlan S (1984) Human T cell growth factor: partial amino acid sequence, cDNA cloning and organization and expression in normal and leukemic cells. Proc Natl Acad Sci USA 81:2543-2547.

Clark SC, Kamen R (1987) The human hematopoietic colony-stimulating factors. Science 236:1229-1237.

Cline MJ, Golde DW (1974) Production of colony stimulating activity by human lymphocytes. Nature 248:703-704.

Clutterbuck EJ, Sanderson CJ (1988) Human eosinophil hematopoiesis studied in vitro by means of murine eosinophil differentiation factor (IL-5): Production of functionally active eosinophils from normal human bone marrow. Blood 71:646-651.

Dinarello CA (1984) Interleukin-1. Rev Infect Dis 6:51.

Dispersio J, Billing P, Kaufman S, Naccache P, Borgeat P, Gasson J (1987) The human GM-CSF receptor: Mechanisms of transmembrane signalling and neutrophil priming. Blood 70:170a (abstract).

Dexter TM, Allen TD, Lajtha LG (1977) Conditions controlling the proliferation of hematopoietic stem cells in vitro. J Cell Physiol 91:335.

Doukas MA, Niskanen E, Quesenberry PJ (1985) Lithium stimulation of granulopoiesis in diffusion chambers-a model of humoral, indirect stimulation of stem cell proliferation. Blood 65:163-168.

Fleischmann J, Golde DW, WEisbart RH, Gasson JC (1986) Granulocyte macrophage colony stimulating factor enhances phagocytosis of bacteria by human neutrophils. Blood 68:708-711.

Friedenstein AF, Chailakhjan RK, Lalykina KS (1970) The development of fibroblast colonies in nonlayer cultures of guinea-pig marrow and spleen cells. Cell Tissue Kinet 3:393.

Ganser A, Volkers B, Greher J, Ottmann Og, Walther F, Becher R, Bergman L, Schulz G, Hoelzer D (1989) Recombinant human granulocyte-macrophage colony stimulating factor in patients with myelodysplastic syndromes - a Phase I/II trial. Blood 73:31-37.

Gasson JC, Weisbart RH, Kaufman SE, Clark SC, Hewick RM, Wong GG, Golde DW (1984) Purified human granulocyte-macrophage colony stimulating factor: direct action on neutrophils. Science 226:1339-1342.

Golde DW, Cline MJ (1972) Identification of the colony stimulating cell in human peripheral blood. J Clin Invest 51:2981-2983.

Gordon MY, Riley GP, Watt SM, Geaves MF (1987) Compartmentalization of a hematopoietic growth factor (GM-CSF) by glycosaminoglycans in the bone marrow microenvironment. Nature 326:403.

Greenberger JS (1978) Sensitivity of corticosteroid dependent insulin-resistant lipogeneses in marrow preadipocytes of obese diabetic (db/db) mice. Nature (London) 275:752.

Gualtieri RJ, Shadduck R, Baker DG, Quesenberry PJ (1984) Hematopoietic regulatory factors produced in long term bone marrow cultures and the effect of in vitro irradiation. Blood 64:516-525.

Guez M, Sachs L (1973) Purification of the protein that induces cell differentiation to macrophages and granulocytes. FEBS Lett 37:149-154.

Hamilton JA, Vairo G, Lingelbach SR (1986) SCF-1 stimulates glucose uptake in murine bone marrow-derived macrophages. Biochem Biophys Res Comm 138:445-454.

Handman E, Burgess AW (1979) Stimulation by granulocyte-macrophage colony stimulating factor of Leishmania tropica killing by macrophages. J Immunol 122:1134-1137.

Hirano T, Taga T, Nakano N, Yasukawa K, Kashiwamura S, Shimizu K, Nakajima K, Pyun KH, Kishimoto T (1985) Purification to homogeneity and characterization of human B cell differentiation factor (BCDF or BSFp-2). Proc Natl Acad Sci USA 82:5490-5494.

Hirano T, Yasukawa K, Harada H, Taga T, Watanabe Y, Matsudaa T, Kashiwarmura S, Nakajima K, Koyama K, Iwamatsu A (1986) Complementary DNA for a novel human interleukin (BSF-2) that induces B lymphocytes to produce immunoglobulin. Nature 324:73-76.

Horiguchi J, Warren MK, Kufe D (1987) Expression of the macrophage-specific colony stimulating factor in human monocytes treated with granulocyte/macrophage colony stimulating factor. Blood 69:1259-1261.

Ihle JN, Keller J, Henderson L et al (1982) Procedures of the purification of IL-3 to homogeneity. J Immunol 129:2431.

Ihle JN, Keller J, Oroszlan S, Henderson LE, Copeland TD, Fitch F, Prystowsky MB, Goldwasser E, Schrader JW, Palaszynski E, Dy M, Lebel B (1983) Biochemical and biological properties of interleukin-3: A lymphokine mediating the differentiation of a lineage of cells which includes prothymocytes and mast-like cells. J Immunol 131:282-287.

Ikebuchi K, Wong GG, Clark SC, Ihle JN, Hirai Y, Ogawa M (1987) Interleukin-6 enhancement of interleukin-3 dependent proliferation of multipotential hemopoietic progenitors. Proc Natl Acad Sci USA 84:9035-9039.

Ikebuchi K, Ihle JN, Hirai Y, Wong GG, Clark SC, Ogawa M (1988) Synergistic factors for stem cell proliferation: Further studies of the target stem cells and the mechanism of stimulation by interleukin-1, interleukin-6 and granulocyte colony stimulating factor. Blood 72:2007-2014.

Jubinsky PT, Stanley Er (1985) Purification of hemopoietin 1: A multilineage hemopoietic growth factor. Proc Natl Acad Sci USA 82:2764-2768.

Karbassi A, Becker JM, Foster JS, Moore RN (1989) Enhanced killing of candida albicons by murine macrophages treated with macrophage colony stimulating factor: Evidence for augmented expression of mannose receptors. J Immunol 139:417-421.

Kaushansky K, Broudy VC, HArlan JM, Adamson JW (1987) Tumor necrosis factor (TNF-alpha) and lymphotoxin (TNF-beta) stimulate the production of GM-CSF, M-CSF, and IL-1 production in vivo. Blood 70:174a (abstract).

Kawano M, Hirano T, Matsuda T, Taga T, Horii Y, Iwato K, Asaoku H, Tang B, Tanabe O, Tanaka H, Kutamoto A, Kishimoto T (1988) Autocrine generation and essential requirement of BSF-2/IL-6 for human multiple myeloma. Nature 332:83-85.

Kinashi T, Harada N, Severinson E, Tanabe T, Sideras P, Knoishi M, Azuma C, Tominaga A, Bergstedt-Linquist S, Takahashi M (1986) Cloning of complementary DNA encoding T cell replacing factor and identity with B cell growth factor II. Nature 324:70-73.

Knudtzon S, Mortensen BI (1975) Growth stimulation of human bone marrow cells in agar culture by vascular cells. Blood 46:937-943.

Koeffler HP, Gasson J, Ranyard J, Souza L, Shepard M, Munker R (1987) Recombinant human TNF stimulates production of granulocyte colony stimulating factor. Blood 70:55-59.

Le PT, Kuetzberg J, Brandt SJ, Niedel JE, Haynes BF, Singer KH (1988) Human thymic epithelial cells produce granulocytes and macrophage colony stimulating factors. J Immunol 141:1211-1217.

Lee F, Yokota T, Otsuka T, Meyerson P, Villaret D, Coffman R, Mosmann T, Rennick D, Roehm N, Smith C (1986) Isolation and characterization of a mouse cDNA clone that expresses B cell stimulatory factor-1 activities and T-cell and mast-cell-stimulating activities. Proc Natl Acad Sci USA 83:2061-2065.

Lin HS, Gordon S (1979) Secretion of plasminogen activator by bone marrow derived mononuclear phagocytes and its enhancement by colony stimulating factor. J Exp Med 150:231-245.

Lovhaug D, Pelus LM, Nordlie EM, Boyum A, Moore MAS (1986) Monocyte-conditioned medium and interleukin 1 induce granulocyte macrophage colony stimulating factor production in the adherent layer of murine bone marrow cultures. Exp Hematol 14:1037-1042.

March CJ, Mosley B, Larsen A, Cerretti DP, Braedt G, Price V, Gillis S, Henney CS, Kronheim SR, Grabstein K, Conlon PJ, Hopp TP, Cosman D (1985) Cloning, sequence and expression of two distinct human interleukin-1 complementary DNAs. Nature 315:641-647.

May LT, Helfgott DC, Sehgal PB (1986) Anti-B-interferon antibodies inhibit the increased expression of HLA-B7 mRNA in tumor necrosis factor-treated human fibroblasts: structural studies of the B2-interferon involved. Proc Natl Acad Sci USA 83:895.

McGrath HE, Liang C, Alberico T, Quesenberry PJ (1987) The effect of lithium on growth factor production in long term bone marrow cultures. Blood 70:1136-1142.

McGrath E, McNiece I, Robinson B, Quesenberry PJ (1989) Unpublished data.

McNiece IK, Bradley TR, Kriegler AB, Hodgson GS (1982) A growth factor produced by WEHI-3 cells for murine high proliferative potential GM-progenitor colony forming cells. Cell Biol Int Rep 6:243.

McNiece IK, McGrath HE, Quesenberry PJ (1988a) Granulocyte colony stimulating factor augments in vitro megakaryocyte colony formation by Interleukin-3. Exp Hematol 16:807-810.

McNiece IK, Robinson BE, Quesenberry PJ (1988b) Stimulation of murine colony forming cells with high proliferative potential by the combination of GM-SCF and SCF-1. Blood 72:191-195.

McNiece IK, Stewart FM, Deacon DH, Quesenberry PJ (1988c) Synergistic interactions between hematopoietic growth factors as detected by in vitro mouse bone marrow colony formation. Exp Hematol 16:383-388.

Metcalf D, Nicola NA (1985) Synthesis by mouse peritoneal cells of granulocyte-colony stimulating factor, the differentiation inducer for myeloid leukemia cells: Stimulation by endotoxin, macrophage colony stimulating factor and multi-colony stimulating factor. Leukemia Res 9:35-50.

Metcalf D, Begley CG, Johnson GR, Nicola NA, Vadas MA, Lopez AF, Williamson DJ, Wong GG, Clark SC, Wang EA (1986) Biologic properties in vitro of a recombinant human granulocyte-macrophage colony stimulating factor. Blood 67:37-45.

Metcalf D, Burgess AW, Johnson GR, Nicola NA, Nice EC, DeLamarter J, Thatcher DR, Mermod J-J (1986) In vitro actions on hemopoietic cells of recombinant murine GM-CSF purified after production in Escherichia coli: comparison with purified native GM-CSF. J Cell Physiol 128:421-431.

Miyauchi J, Kelleher CA, Yang Y-C, Wong GG, Clark SC, Minden MD, Minkin S, McCulloch EA (1987) The effects of three recombinant growth factors IL-3, GM-CSF and G-CSF on the blast cells of acute myeloblastic leukemia maintained in short term suspension culture. Blood 70: 657-663.

Mochizuki DY, Eisenman JR, Conlon PJ, Larson AD, Tuckinski RS (1987) Interleukin-1 regulates hematopoietic activity, a role previously ascribed to hemopoietin 1. Proc Natl Acad Sci USA 84:5267-5271.

Moore MAS, Williams N (1972) Physical separation of colony stimulating cells from in vitro colony forming cells in hemopoietic tissues. J Cell Physiol 80:195-206.

Morgan DA, Ruscetti FW, Gallo RC (1976) Selective in vitro growth of T lymphocytes from normal human bone marrow. Science 193:1007-1008.

Munker R, Gasson J, Ogawa M, Koeffler HP (1986) Recombinant human TNF induces production of granulocyte-monocyte colony stimulating factor. Nature 232:79-82.

Namen AE, Lupton S, Hjerrild K, Wignall J, Mochizuki DY, Schmierer A, Moslely B, March CJ, Urdal D, Gillis S (1988a) Stimulation of B cell progenitors by cloned murine interleukin-7. Nature 333:571-573.

Namen AE, Schmierer AE, March CJ, Overall RW, Park LS, Urdal DL, Mochizuki DY (1988b) B cell precursor growth-promoting activity. Purification and characterization of a growth factor active on lymphocyte precursors. J Exp Med 167:988-1002.

Namen AE: Presented at American Red Cross meeting, Washington, DC, 1989.

Nicola NA, Metcalf D, Matsumoto M, Johnson GR (1983) Purification of a factor inducing differentiation in murine myelomonocytic leukemia cells. Identification as granulocyte colony stimulating factor. J Biol Chem 258:9017-9023.

Nicola NA, Begley CG, Metcalf D (1985) Identification of the human analogue of a regulator that induces differentiation in murine leukaemic cells. Nature 314:625-628.

Noma Y, Sideras P, Naito T, Bergstedt-Linquist S, Azuma C, Severinson E, Tanabe T, Kinashi T, Matsuda F, Yaoita Y (1986) Cloning of cDNA encoding the murine IgGl induction factor by a novel strategy using SP6 promoter. Nature 319:640-646.

Oster W, Lindemann A, Horn S, Mertelmann R, Herrmann F (1987) Tumor necrosis factor (TNF)-alpha but not TNF beta induces secretion of colony stimulating factor for macrophages (CSF-2) by human monocytes. Blood 70:1700-1703.

Parker JW, Metcalf D (1974) Production of colony stimulating factor in mitogen stimulated lymphocyte cultures. J Immunol 112:502-510.

Peschel C, Paul WE, Ohara J, Green I (1987) Effects of B cell stimulatory factor-1 (interleukin-4) on hematopoietic progenitor cells. Blood 70:254.

Prystowsky MB, Ihle JN, Rich I, et al (1983) Two biologically distinct colony stimulating factors are secreted by a T lymphocyte clone. J Cell Biochem 6:37.

Quesenberry P, Levitt L (1979) Hematopoietic stem cells. N Engl J Med Part I 301:755-760; Part II 301:819--823; Part III 301:868-872.

Quesenberry P, Gimbrone M (1980) Vascular endothelium as a regulator of granulopoieses: Production of colony stimulating activity by cultured human endothelial cells. Blood 56:1060-1067.

Quesenberry PJ, Gimbrone MA, Doukas MA, Goldwasser E (1981) Vascular derived tissues as a source of colony stimulating activity (CSA). Clin Res 29:830a (abstract).

Quesenberry PJ, Gimbrone M (1983) Synthesis of colony-stimulating activity of endothelial cells. In: The Biology of Endothelial Cells, edited by EA Jaffe. Vol. 27. Martinus Nijjjhoff, Netherlands.

Quesenberry PJ, Ihle JN, McGrath E (1985) The effect of interleukin-3 and GM-CSA-2 on megakaryocyte and myeloid clonal colony formation. Blood 65:214-217.

Quesenberry P, Song Z, McGrath H, McNiece I, Shadduck R, Waheed A, Baber G, Kleeman E, Kaiser D (1987) Multilineage synergistic activity produced by a murine adherent marrow cell line. Blood 69:827-835.

Quesenberry P: unpublished observations, 1988.

Ramaldi A, Young DC, Griffin JD (1987) Expression of the macrophage-colony stimulating factor (CSF-1) gene by human monocytes. Blood 69:1409-1413.

Rennick D, Yang G, Muller-Sieburg C, Smith C, Arai N, Takabe Y, Gemmell L (1987) Interleukin 4 (B cell stimulatory factor-1) can enhance or antagonize the factor dependent growth of hematopoietic progenitor cells. Proc Natl Acad SCi USA 84:6889.

Robinson BE, McGrath HE, Quesenberry PJ (1987) Recombinant murine granulocyte macrophage colony stimulating factor has megakaryocyte colony stimulating activity and augments megakaryocyte colony stimulation by interleukin-3. J Clin Invest 79:1648-1652.

Sanderson CJ, Warren DJ, Strath M (1985) Identification of a lymphokine that stimulates differentiation in vitro. Its relationship to interleukin-3 and functional properties of the eosinophils produced in cultures. J Exp Med 162:60.

Sanderson C: presented at WEHI meeting, Melbourne, Australia, 1988.

Schimpl A, Wecker E (1972) Replacement of T cell function by a T cell product. Nature 237:15.

Sieff CA, Emerson SG, Donahue RE, Nathan DG (1985) Human recombinant granulocyte-macrophage colony stimulating factor: a multilineage hematopoietin. Science 230:1171-1173.

Silberstein DS, Owen WF, Gasson JC, DiPersio JF, Golde DW, Bina JC, Soberman R, Austen KF, David JR (1986) Enhancement of human eosinophil cytotoxicty and leukotriene synthesis by biosynthetic (recombinant) granulocyte-macrophage colony stimulating factor. J Immunol 137:3290-3294.

Song ZX, Quesenberry PJ (1984) Radioresistant murine marrow stromal cells: a morphologic and functional characterization. Exp Hematol 12:523-533.

Stanley ER, Heard PM (1977) Factors regulating macrophage production and growth. Purification and some properties of the colony stimulating factor from medium. J Biol Chem 252:4305-4312.

Stanley ER, Guilbert LF (1981) Methods of purification, assay, characterization and target cell binding of a colony-stimulating factor (CSF-1). J Immunol Meth 42:253-284.

Stanley E, Burgess AW (1983) Granulocyte macrophage colony stimulating factor stimulates the synthesis of membrane and nuclear proteins in murine neutophils. J Cell Biochem 23:241-258.

Stanley ER, Jubinsky PT (1984) Factors affecting the growth and differentiation of hemopoietic cells in culture. Clin Hematol 13:329.

Swain SL, Dutton RW (1982) Production of a B cell growth promoting activity, (DL) BCGF, from a cloned T cell line and its assay on the BCL1 B cell tumor. J Exp Med 156:1821.

Takatsu K, Tominaga A, Mamaoka T (1980) Antigen induced T cell replacing factor (TRF). I. Functional characterization of TRF-producing helper T cell subset and genetic studies on TRF production. J Immunol 124:2414.

Tanabe O, Akira S, Kamiya aT, Wong GG, Hirano T, Kishimoto T (1988) Genomic structure of the murine IL-6 gene. High degree conservation of potential regulatory sequences between mouse and human. J Immunol 141:3875-3881.

Testa NG, Dexter TM (1977) Long term production of erythroid precursor cells (BFU) in bone marrow cultures. Differentiation 9:193.

Vadas MA, Nicola NA, Metcalf D (1983) Activation of antibody dependent cell mediated cytotoxicity of the human neutrophils and eosinophils by separate colony stimulating factors. J Immunol 130:795-799.

Vallenga E, Young DC, Wagner K, Wiper D, Ostapovicz D, Griffin JD (1987) The effects of GM-CSF and G-CSF in promoting gr owth of clonogenic cells in acute myeloblastic leukemia. Blood 69:1771-1776.

Van Damme J, Openakker G, Simpson RJ, Rubira MR, Cayphas S, Vink A, Billior A, van Snick J (1987) Identification of the human 26-kd protein, interferon B2 (IFN-B2) as a B cell hybridoma/plasmacytoma growth factor induced by interleukin-1 and tumor necrosis factor. J Exp Med 165:914.

Waheed A, Shadduck RF (1979) Purification and properties of L cell-derived colony-stimulating factor. J Lab Clin Med 94: 180-194.

Wang JM, Chen ZG, Colella S, Bonilla MA, Welte K, Bordignon C, Mantovani A (1988) Chemotactic activity of recombinant human granulocyte colony-stimulating factor. Blood 72:1456-1460.

Weisbart RH, Golde DW, Clark SC, Wong G-G, Jasson JC (1985) Human granulocyte-macorphage colony stimulating factor is a neutrophil activator. Nature 314:361-363.

Williams NH, Jackson H, Rabellino EM (1977) Proliferation and differentiation of normal granulopoietic cells in continuous bone marrow cultures. J Cell Physiol 93:435.

Williams NH, Jackson H, Sheridan APC et al (1978) Regulation of megakaryopoiesis in long-term murine bone marrow cultures. Blood 51:245.

Wing EJ, Waheed A, Shadduck RK, Nagle LS, Stephenson K (1982) Effect of colony stimulating factor on murine macrophages. J Clin Invest 69:270-276.

Wing EJ, Ampel NM, Waheed A, Shadduck RK (1985) Macrophage CSF (M-CSF) enhances the capacity of murine macrophages to secrete oxygen reduction products. J Immunol 135:2052-2056.

Wong GG, Golde DW (1984) Purified human granulocyte-macrophage colony stimulating factor: direct action on neutrophils. Science 226:1339-1342.

Wong GG, Witck-Giannotti JS, Temple PA, Kriz R, Ferenz C, Hewick RM, Clark SC, Ikebuchi K, Ogawa M (1988) Stimulation of murine hemopoietic colony formation by human IL-6. J Immunol 140:3040-3044.

Yang Y-C, Ciarletta AB, Temple PA et al (1986) Human interleukin-3 (multi-CSF): Identification by expression cloning of a novel hematopoietic growth factor related to murine interleukin-3. Cell 47:3.

Yokota T, Lee F, Rennick D, Hall C, Arai N, Mosmann T, Nabel G, Cantor H, Arai K (1984) Isolation and characterization of a mouse cDNA clone that expresses ast cell growth factor activity in monkey cells. Proc Natl Acad Sci USA 81:1070-1074.

Ziboh VA, Miller AM, Wu M-C, Yunis AA, Jimenez J, Wong G (1982) Induced release and metabolism of arachidonic acid from myeloid cells by purified colony stimulating factor. J Cell Physiol 113:67-72.

Zilberstein A, Ruggieri R, Korn JH, Revel M (1986) Structure and expression of cDNA and genes for human interferon B-2, a distinct species inducible by growth stimulatory cytokines. Embo J 5:2529-2537.

Zucali JR, Dinarello CA, Oblon DF, Gross MA, Anderson L, Weiner RS, (1986) Interleukin 1 stimulates fibroblasts to produce granulocyte-macrophage colony stimulating activity and porstaglandin E2. J Clin Invest 77:1857-1863.

Hematopoietic Growth Factors
in Transfusion Medicine, pages 19–26

ERYTHROPOIETIN: MOLECULAR AND CELLULAR BIOLOGY

Eugene Goldwasser

Department of Biochemistry and Molecular Biology, The University of Chicago, Chicago, Illinois 60637

INTRODUCTION

The study of the control of red cell formation, as a model of the more general process of cell differentiation, offers many advantages for an experimentalist. Not only is the mature red cell well characterized but the mechanisms that control the rate of erythrocyte production, are beginning to be understood. The normal steady-state rate of formation of about 2.5 million red cells per second in man can increase up to about 17 million per second under anemic or hypoxic stress. An increase in circulating red cells, as for instance by transfusion or exposure for some time to low oxygen, results in decreased red cell production. The normal, accelerated and decreased rates all appear to be controlled by the glycoprotein, erythropoietin (epo). As first proposed more than 80 years (Carnot, 1906) but on evidence that is not precisely duplicable, there is a homeostatic mechanism by which a fall in oxygen carrying capacity causes a signal that, in turn, causes a rise in circulating red cells. This signal, epo, is a glycoprotein of molecular size 30,400 with about 39% carbohydrate (Davis et al., 1987).

RESULTS

Human urinary epo (Miyake et al., 1977) has a specific activity (units per mg of protein) of about 80 - 100,000 whereas purified human recombinant epo has a potency of about 160 - 180,000. This discrepancy may be due to a conformational difference and is still under study. Using 129,000 U/mg as the potency of fully glycsoylated epo, one unit is about 7.75 ng of epo or 0.255 p moles. The radioimmunoassay and the bone marrow culture assay can detect epo in the mU range; 1 mU is equivalent to 154 million molecules.

The use of molecular biological techniques has yielded important data about the properties of epo (Jacobs, et al., 1985; Lin et al., 1985; McDonald et al., 1986; Shoemaker and Mistock, 1986). There is a single copy epo gene consisting of five exons and four introns. The human epo gene encodes a protein of 193 amino acid residues including the initiator methionine. Twenty-seven of these residues form a leader sequence and 166 residues are in the mature protein. The C-terminal arginine is probably cleaved by a circulating protease (Recny et al., 1987). For the monkey (genus Macaca) the leader sequence also has 27 residues but the mature protein has 165 residues, lacking the lysine at position 116 (Lin et al., 1986). In the mouse the leader sequence has 26 residues and the mature protein 166 (McDonald et al., 1986; Shoemaker and Mistock, 1986).

The human and monkey sequences (not considering the leader) have 151 residues that are identical, one residue 116, is lacking in the monkey and of the remaining 14, seven amino acid replacements are conservative. Similarly the mouse and human sequences have 135 residues identical (80%). Of the remaining 31, 18 of the replacements are conservative. The three asparagine residues, 24, 38, and 83, that are glycosylation sites are conserved in all three species. The O-linked glycosylation site (serine 126 in human) also exists in monkey at position 125, but is replaced by a proline in the mouse.

Human epo has two disulfide bonds bridging residues 7 and 161 and 29 and 33. Maintenance of one or both of these is essential for biological activity. If epo is reduced, denatured, renatured and re-oxidized, essentially all of the biological action is restored (Wang et al., 1985).

The structures of the sialic acid terminal oligosaccharides of human epo have been determined (Sasaki et al., 1987; Takeuchi et al., 1988). Sialic acid termini are essential for <u>in vivo</u> stability but not for intrinsic biological activity i.e. the effect on epo-responsive cells (Goldwasser et al., 1974). Removal of the oligosaccharide chains results in loss of in vivo activity accompanied by extensive aggregation, but small amount of non-aggregated aglyco-epo remaining has increased intrinsic activity (Dordal et al., 1985).

Very little is known about the structural features of the polypeptide required for biological activity. Data on site-directed mutagenesis indicate that replacement in human epo of systeine 33 by proline, as in the case in mouse epo, results in loss of activity (Lin, 1987).

Cloning and expression of the epo gene in commercial quantities has made possible the successful use in treatment of some anemias (Eschbach et al., 1987; Winearls et al., 1986). It has also provided a deeper understanding of some aspects of epo biology. The single copy gene on human chromosome 7 (7pter - ->q11 - 22) (Law et al., 1986; Watkins et al., 1986) or mouse chromosome 5 (Lacombe et al., 1988) consists of five exons separated by four introns. The DNA sequences of human, monkey and mouse shows that intron length except for the first intron, is not well conserved. With respect to sequence, the 10-20 bases at the intron-exon boundaries are moderately well conserved; the remainder shows essentially no homology. The coding sequences show 94% identity between human and monkey and 79% identity between human and mouse. With respect to both DNA and protein, epo has been highly conserved in the period since the mammalian radiation (about 200 million years).

More than thirty years ago the organ of origin of epo was found to be the adult kidney (Jacobson et al., 1957) but the evidence was not conclusive since it permitted other, more complex, interpretations. Molecular hybridization methods showed conclusively that the adult kidney was a source of epo (Beru et al., 1986; Bondurant and Koury, 1986) and that epo mRNA was not detected by the conventional Northern technique in any other organ, with occasional exception of the liver (Beru et al., 1986). Since there is evidence that fetal liver can produce epo (Zanjani et al., 1977) it is possible that the developmental mechanism that causes the switch from fetal liver to adult kidney can be reversed, under conditions of severe hypoxic stress to the adult.

The question of which cells in the kidney respond to hypoxia by synthesis and secretion of epo is, in principle, answerable by the *in situ* hybridization method, which localizes specific mRNA species. Published results indicate that epo is made by a sub-population of interstitial cells of the renal cortex (Koury et al., 1987; Lacombe et al., 1987); unpublished results from this laboratory, using the same general method indicate, that the cells of origin are in a sub-population of proximal tubule cells. This problem needs further study.

The mechanism by which the cells respond to oxygen lack has begun to be understood, by use of a hepatoma cell line that secretes epo in response to hypoxia or cobalt salts (Goldberg et al., 1988). The data strongly suggest that a heme protein is involved in the signal transduction between the hypoxic environment and the expression of the epo gene.

In our own studies of the molecular mechanism regulating expression of the epo gene, N. Beru has found evidence, by the gel retardation method, for the involvement of a DNA binding protein, specific for a 17 base sequence upstream of the transcription start site of the mouse gene. When kidneys from mice after hypoxia or cobalt salt administration are compared with untreated kidneys, extracts of nuclei from kidneys of treated mice show a greatly reduced label of a protein that binds specifically to the 17 mer. This protein is approximately 24 kda in size and may be a negative transcription factor, so that response of the epo gene to hypoxia may depend on loss of this protein or its modification to a non-binding form.

Study of transformed cells that express the epo gene constitutively indicate that one line of these cells (IW32) (Tambourin et al., 1983) has an amplified and rearranged epo gene as well as a normal epo gene (McDonald et al., 1987). We have found, by sequencing the upstream region of the rearranged gene, an expressed gene on the complementary strand. This "new" gene appears to have caused epo gene expression because of the adventitious translocation of the epo gene to close proximity of the "new" gene (Beru et al., 1989).

Once epo is secreted it is delivered to target cells by circulation. There is continuum of cells in the bone marrow that are affected by epo, but one requirement for all of these cells must be the presence of specific receptors for epo. Although receptor presence was inferred from experiments with impure epo and impure cells (Chang et al., 1974), it could have been inferred simply from the fact that epo has biological activity. The first quantitative study of receptors was made possible by having pure, labelled epo and a pure population of epo-responsive cells (Krantz and Goldwasser, 1984). Because of the possibility that high specific activity iodinated epo might be biologically inactive, these earlier experiments were done with tritiated epo and were limited by low specific activity. When it was found that iodinated epo could bind to target cells specifically, regardless of biological activity, the problem was studied with greater precision and sensitivity. The results showed a small number of specific epo receptors with two classes of affinity constants. The higher affinity receptors (k_D = 90 pM) appear to be the biologically relevant ones (Sawyer et al., 1987).

The method of expression cloning was used to isolate and characterize a cDNA clone for the mouse epo receptor. (D'Andrea et al., 1989). From the cDNA structure it was deduced that the epo receptor is a protein of 507 amino acid residues; with a 23 residue leader sequence, an extracellular domain, a membrane-spanning domain, and a C-terminal cytoplasmic domain. When this single copy gene is expressed in COS cells there are generated receptors with both low and high affinity as in those findings described earlier. This apparent paradox still needs resolution.

The experiments from this laboratory were performed under grants No. HL21676 and HL 30121 from the National Heart, Lung, and Blood Institute, N.I.H.

REFERENCES

Beru N, McDonald J, Lacombe C, Goldwasser E (1986). Expression of the erythropoietin gene. Mol Cell Biol 6:2571-2575.

Beru N, McDonald J, Goldwasser E (1989).Activation of the erythropoietin gene due to the proximity of an expressed gene. DNA 8:253-259.

Bondurant MC, Koury MJ (1986). Anemia induces accumulation of erythropoietin mRNA in the kidney and lever. Mol Cell Biol 6:2731-2733.

Carnot P (1906). Sur le mecanisme d 'hyperglobulie provoquee par le serum d'animaux en renovation sanguine. CR Acad Scie (Paris) 111:344-346.
Chang SC-S, Sikkema D, Goldwasser E (1974). Evidence for an erythropoietin receptor protein on rat bone marrow cells. Biochem Biophys Res Commun 57:339-405.
D'Andrea AD, Lodish HF, Wong GG (1989). Expression cloning of the murine erythropoietin receptor. Cell 57:277-285.
Davis JM, Arakawa T, Strickland TW, Yphantis DA (1987). Characterization of recombinant human erythropoietin produced in Chinese hamster ovary cells. Biochem 26:2633-2638.
Dordal MS, Wang FF, Goldwasser E (1985). The role of carbohydrate in erythropoietin action. Endocrinol 116:2293-2299.
Eschbach JW, Egrie JC, Downing MR, Browne JK, Adamson JW (1987). Correction of the anemia of end-stage renal disease with recombinant human erythropoietin. New Eng J Med 316:73-77.
Goldberg MA, Dunning SP, Bunn HF (1988). Regulation of the erythropoietin gene: Evidence that the oxygen sensor is a heme protein. Science 242:1412-1415.
Goldwasser E, Kung CK-H, Eliason JF (1974). On the mechanism of erythropoietin induced differentiation. XIII The role of sialic acid in erythro poietin action. J Biol Chem 249:4202-4206.
Jacobs K, Shoemaker C, Rudersdorf R, Neill SD, Kaufman RJ, Mufson A, Seehra H, Jones SS, Hewick R, Fritsch EF, Kawakita M, Shimizu T, Miyake T (1985). Isolation and characterization of genomic and cDNA clones of human erythropoietin. Nature 313:806-810.
Jacobson LO, Goldwasser E, Fried W, Plzak LF (1957). Role of the kidney in erythropoiesis. Nature 179:633-634.
Koury ST, Bondurant MC, Koury MJ (1987). Localization of erythropoietin synthesizing cells in murine kidneys by in situ hybridization. Blood 71:524-527.
Krantz SB, Goldwasser E (1984). Specific binding of erythropoietin to spleen cells infected with anemia strain of Friend virus. Proc Natl Acad Sci (USA) 81:7574-7578.
Lacombe C, Da Silva JL, Bruneval P, Fournier J-G, Wendling F, Casadevall N, Camilleri J-P, Bariety J, Varet B, Tambourin P (1987). Pertibular cells are the site of erythropoietin synthesis in the murine hypoxic

kidney. J Clin Invest 81:620-623.
Lacombe C, Tambourin P, Mattei MG, Simon D, Guenet JL (1988). The murine erythropoietin gene is localized on chromosome 5. Blood 72:1440-1442.
Law ML, Cai G-Y, Lin F-K, Wei Q, Huang S-Z, Hartz JH, Morse H, Lin C-H, Jones C, Kao F-T (1986). Chromosomal assignment of the human erythropoietin gene and its DNA polymorphism. Proc Natl Acad Scie (USA) 83:6920-6924.
Lin FK, Suggs S, Lin CH, Browne J, Smalling R, Egrie J, Chen K, Fox G, Martin F, Stabinsky Z, Badrawi S, Lai PH, Goldwasser E (1985). Cloning and expression of the human erythropoietin gene. Proc Natl Acad Sci (USA) 82:7580-7584.
Lin FK, Line C-H, Lai P-H, Browne JK, Egrie JC, Smalling R, Fox GM, Chen KK, Castro M, Suggs S (1986). Monkey erythropoietin gene: Cloning, expression and comparison with the human erythropoietin gene. Gene 44:201-209.
Lin FK (1987). The molecular biology of erythropoietin. In Rich IN (ed): "Molecular and Cellular Aspects of Erythropoietin and Erythropoiesis," Berlin: Springer Verlag, pp 23-26.
McDonald J, Lin FK, Goldwasser E (1986). Cloning, sequencing and evolutionary analysis of the mouse erythropoietin gene. Mol Cell Biol 6:842-848.
McDonald J, Beru N, Goldwasser E (1987). Rearrangement and expression of erythropoietin genes in transformed mouse cells. Mol Cell Biol 7:365-370.
Miyake T, Kung CK-H, Goldwasser E (1977). Purification of human erythropoietin. J Biol Chem 252:5558-5564.
Recny MA, Scoble HA, Kim Y (1987). Structural characterization of natural human urinary and recombinant DNA-derived erythropoietin, J Biol Chem 262:17156-17163.
Sasaki H, Bothner B, Dell A, Fukuda M (1987). Carbohydrate structure of erythrpoietin expressed in Chinese hamster ovary cells by a human erythropoietin cDNA. J Biol Chem 262:12059-12076.
Sawyer ST, Krantz SB, Goldwasser E (1987). Binding and receptor-mediated endocytosis of erythropoietin in Friend virus-infected erythroid cells. J Biol Chem 262:5554-5562.

Shoemaker CB, Mistock LD (1986). Murine erythropoietin gene: Cloning, expression, and human gene homology. Mol Cell Biol 6:849-858.

Takeuchi M, Takasaki S, Miyazaki H, Kato T, Hoshi S, Kochibe N, Kobata A (1988). Comparative study of the asparagine-linked sugar chains of human erythropoietin purified from urine and the culture medium of recombinant Chinese hamster ovary cells. J Biol Chem 263:3657-3663.

Wang FF, Kung CK-H, Goldwasser E (1985). Some chemical properties of human erythropoietin. Endocrinol 116:2286-2292.

Watkins, PC, Eddy R, Hoffman N, Stanislovitis P, Beck AK, Galli J, Vellucci V, Gusella JF, SHows TB (1986). Regional chromosome region 7pter - ->q22. Cell Genet 42:214-218.

Winearls CG, Oliver DO, Pippard MJ, Reid C, Downing MR, Cotes PM (1986). Effect of human erythropoietin derived from recombinant DNA on the anaemia of patients maintained by chronic hemodialysis. Lancet 2:1175-1177.

Zanjani ED, Foster I, Burlington H, Wasserman LR (1977). Liver as the primary site erythropoietin formation in the fetus. J Lab Clin Med 89:640-644.

Hematopoietic Growth Factors
in Transfusion Medicine, pages 27–41

HUMAN GRANULOCYTE-MACROPHAGE COLONY-STIMULATING FACTOR (GM-CSF): REGULATION OF EXPRESSION

Judith C. Gasson, John K. Fraser, and
Stephen D. Nimer

Division of Hematology-Oncology, Department of Medicine, UCLA School of Medicine, Los Angeles, CA 90024

INTRODUCTION

The development of semi-solid culture systems, which allow the survival and proliferation of bone marrow progenitor cells, made it possible to identify and characterize hematopoietic growth factors from a variety of biological sources. To date, four human colony-stimulating factors (CSFs) have been purified, molecularly cloned, and extensively characterized (Clark and Kamen, 1987; Golde and Gasson, 1988). The names of these factors are derived from the major type(s) of mature hematopoietic cell which is produced *in vitro*. Thus, interleukin 3 (IL-3; multi-CSF) stimulates the formation of colonies consisting of multiple lineages, including neutrophils, monocytes, eosinophils, and erythroid elements. Granulocyte CSF and macrophage CSF (also known as CSF-1) stimulate the formation of colonies consisting primarily of neutrophilic granulocytes or monocytes, respectively. Granulocyte-macrophage CSF (GM-CSF) likewise stimulates the formation of colonies consisting of neutrophilic and eosinophilic granulocytes and monocytes.

Human GM-CSF is a glycoprotein which is heterogeneously glycosylated, yielding a molecular weight in the range of 22-25,000 daltons. It is encoded by a gene of 2.5 kilobases (kb) in length, with three intervening sequences, which has been mapped to the long arm of chromosome 5 (Huebner et al., 1985).

BIOLOGICAL ACTIVITIES OF HUMAN GM-CSF

In addition to its ability to stimulate the formation of myeloid colonies *in vitro* (Tomonaga et al., 1985), GM-CSF is also active as a hematopoietic growth factor *in vivo*, stimulating a dose-dependent increase in neutrophils, eosinophils, and monocytes (Antman et al., 1988; Brandt et al., 1988; Champlin et al., 1989; Groopman et al., 1987; Vadhan-Raj et al., 1987). In addition, GM-CSF has potent activities on mature myeloid effector cells, enhancing multiple differentiated activities (Figure 1) (Baldwin et al., 1988; DiPersio et al., 1988; Naccache et al., 1988; Silberstein, 1986; Weisbart et al., 1985; Weisbart et al., 1986; Weisbart et al., 1987). Because of its ability to act both as a growth factor and to enhance the functional activity of mature cells, a variety of clinical uses for GM-CSF have been proposed and are currently being explored.

Clinical uses for GM-CSF and other hematopoietic growth factors can be categorized into three general groups. The first is to treat bone marrow failure states such as aplastic anemia or congenital neutropenias, and to enhance hematopoietic recovery following bone marrow transplantation (Brandt et al., 1988; Champlin et al., 1989). The second is to augment host defense in immunocompromised states such as AIDS, lymphoproliferative disorders, and perhaps patients with infections associated with burns, diabetes, and alcoholism (Groopman et al., 1987; Vadhan-Raj et al., 1987). The third is to reduce the myelosuppressive effects of chemotherapy or radiotherapy, which will increase the effectiveness and decrease the toxicity of treatment of solid tumors (Antman et al., 1988).

Hematopoietic growth factor therapy will allow larger doses of cytotoxic agents and more frequent administration by decreasing the morbidity of treatment-induced neutropenia. Because of the considerable interest in employing GM-CSF and other hematopoietic growth factors in a variety of clinical settings and the likely physiologic role of these factors in hematopoiesis and host defense, the expression and mechanism of action of hematopoietins is the focus of intense investigation.

Figure 1. Biological Activities of Human GM-CSF

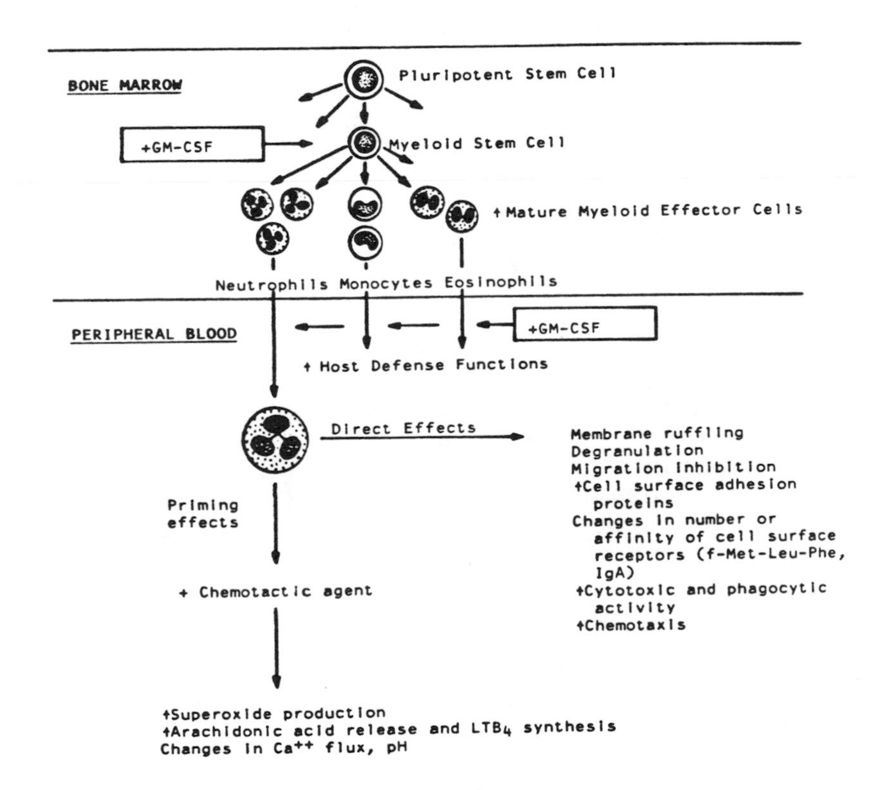

IDENTIFICATION OF CELLS AND TISSUES WHICH EXPRESS GM-CSF

Numerous studies have characterized the cellular sources of human GM-CSF: initially, to identify potential sources of the material for purification, and more recently, to understand the physiologic regulation of GM-CSF production. We and others have shown that T-cells activated by antigen or lectin produce GM-CSF, whereas resting T-cells do not (Chan et al., 1986; Wong et al., 1985). In addition, all human T-cell lines established by infection with HTLV-I or -II constitutively produce GM-CSF. These infected cells also constitutively express the interleukin 2 (IL-2) receptor and other biologically active cytokines. Thus, they mirror the phenotype of an activated T-cell.

GM-CSF can also be produced by certain fibroblasts and endothelial cells stimulated by monokines such as interleukin 1 (IL-1), tumor necrosis factor (TNF), or the potent phorbol ester, TPA (Figure 2) (Bagby et al., 1986; Broudy et al., 1986; Koeffler et al., 1988; Munker et al., 1986). Unlike lymphocytes, in which there is no detectable transcription of the GM-CSF gene prior to activation, nuclear run-on experiments have demonstrated constitutive expression of the GM-CSF gene in unstimulated fibroblasts and endothelial cells but no subsequent accumulation of messenger RNA or protein production. Upon stimulation of the cells by monokines, GM-CSF messenger RNA accumulates, leading to the production of biologically active protein. Nuclear run-on studies have demonstrated small increases in transcription of the gene, and half-life studies have shown greatly increased messenger RNA stability (Koeffler et al., 1988). Thus, the stimulation of GM-CSF production by these cell types is through a combined increase in transcription and stabilization of messenger

RNA. Activated macrophages can also produce GM-CSF through similar mechanisms.

While studies are underway to examine the production of GM-CSF by stromal elements in the bone marrow, such information is currently not available. Therefore, it is difficult to precisely define the role of GM-CSF in homeostatic regulation of hematopoiesis, as well as in response to infection. It is likely that soluble mediators from the periphery could stimulate cells in the bone marrow micro-environment to produce GM-CSF, leading to a subsequent increase in white blood cell count in response to infection. It is not known at this time whether the daily production of neutrophils and monocytes to maintain the normal white blood count is directly controlled by GM-CSF.

Figure 2. Cellular Sources of Human GM-CSF

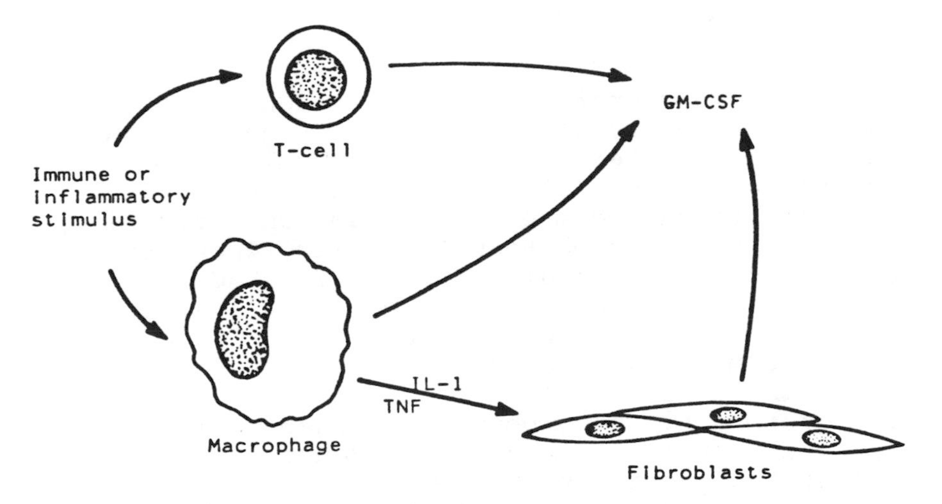

IDENTIFICATION OF SEQUENCES CONTROLLING GM-CSF EXPRESSION

GM-CSF is encoded by a gene 2.5 kb in length, interrupted by three intervening sequences. This gene has been mapped to the long arm of chromosome 5. A number of other growth factor and growth factor receptor genes have been mapped to a relatively small region in the long arm of chromosome 5, including c-fms, the cellular receptor for the macrophage CSF (CSF-1) (Le Beau et al., 1986), and the IL-3 (multi-CSF) gene (Le Beau et al., 1987).

Shaw and Kamen noted an AT-rich region in the 3′ untranslated segment of the GM-CSF gene (Shaw and Kamen, 1986). This motif is found in other cellular genes, including c-*myc*, c-*jun*, and c-*fos*, and was shown to have a destabilizing effect on messenger RNA produced by recombinant constructs. Thus, this region likely plays an important role in GM-CSF messenger RNA turnover.

In order to focus on the promoter elements, we prepared recombinant constructs linking the 5′ region of the GM-CSF gene to the bacterial reporter gene, chloramphenicol acetyltransferase (CAT), to identify the transcriptional control mechanisms important in T-lymphocytes and mesenchymal cells (Chan et al., 1986; Nimer et al., 1988). To study regulation of GM-CSF expression in activated lymphocytes, we chose two T-cell lines which behave similarly to primary T-cells. MLA 144 is a gibbon ape T-cell line which is transformed by the gibbon ape leukemia virus, and constitutively produces IL-2 due to integration of the virus upstream of the IL-2 gene. No constitutive accumulation of GM-CSF messenger RNA can be observed by this cell line using either Northern or S_1 nuclease analyses; however, upon stimulation of the cells with TPA and phytohemagglutinin (PHA), there is a rapid accumulation of GM-CSF messenger RNA within four to six hours, leading to secretion of biologically active protein (Nimer et al., 1988).

We have also examined the human Jurkat T-cell line, which is similar to MLA 144 in that no constitutive expression of GM-CSF messenger RNA can be detected, and there is rapid induction of RNA accumulation after stimulation with TPA and PHA. However, five- to ten-fold lower levels of GM-CSF messenger RNA and protein are produced by this cell line.

Transfection of recombinant constructs containing 626 nucleotides of GM-CSF sequences upstream from the start site of transcription linked to the bacterial CAT gene into either MLA 144 or Jurkat cells does not result in detectable expression of CAT activity in unstimulated cells. Following stimulation of MLA 144 or Jurkat cells by PHA and TPA, there is a thirty- or five-fold enhancement of expression, respectively. A series of 5′ deletion mutants were prepared, the most extensive deletion containing only 53 nucleotides upstream from the start site of transcription. Transfection of these deletion mutants into MLA 144 and Jurkat cells revealed that the level of enhancement observed following mitogen stimulation of cells transfected with constructs containing only 53 nucleotides upstream of the start site was identical to that of the full-length GM-CSF-CAT construct (which contains 626 bp of upstream sequences). Thus, sequences necessary for the expression of GM-CSF in activated T-lymphocyte cell lines appear to be contained within a 90-base pair region containing 53 nucleotides upstream and 37 nucleotides downstream from the cap site (Nimer et al., 1988).

In addition, while the largest promoter construct (-626 nucleotides) did not have constitutive activity in either cell line in the absence of stimulation, a number of the truncated constructs showed constitutive CAT activity in unstimulated Jurkat cells, suggesting the presence of negative regulatory elements in the GM-CSF promoter region. The combined contributions of negative regulatory elements and inducible promoter elements likely play a role in the stimulated transcription of GM-CSF in T-cells.

Biochemical studies were performed to localize the binding of nuclear extract proteins from both stimulated and unstimulated MLA 144 cells to the GM-CSF promoter. The purpose of these studies is to correlate binding of nuclear proteins to regions of the GM-CSF promoter with sequences which are active in directing expression of recombinant constructs in transient transfection experiments. The technique of DNase I footprinting is designed to identify interactions of specific nuclear proteins with promoter sequences. Our results showed that nuclear extracts prepared from MLA 144 cells stimulated with PHA and TPA bound to a specific region in the GM-CSF promoter contained within 53 nucleotides upstream from the start site of transcription (Figure 3) (Nimer et al., 1988). These results strongly support conclusions obtained from the transient transfection studies indicating that this region of the GM-CSF promoter is important in induction of GM-CSF expression in lymphocytes.

We have extended our studies on the sequences regulating GM-CSF expression to human fibroblasts using the WI-38 cell line as a model. Previous work had shown that the GM-CSF gene is constitutively transcribed in certain fibroblasts and endothelial cells; however, messenger RNA and protein do not accumulate unless the cells are stimulated with IL-1, TNF, or phorbol esters. Transfection of recombinant GM-CSF promoter constructs into the fibroblast cell line, WI-38, similarly demonstrated constitutive transcription of these constructs.

GM-CSF promoter sequences located between -53 and +37 can direct the full constitutive expression of these recombinant plasmids (Nimer et al., 1989).

Figure 3. Human GM-CSF Gene

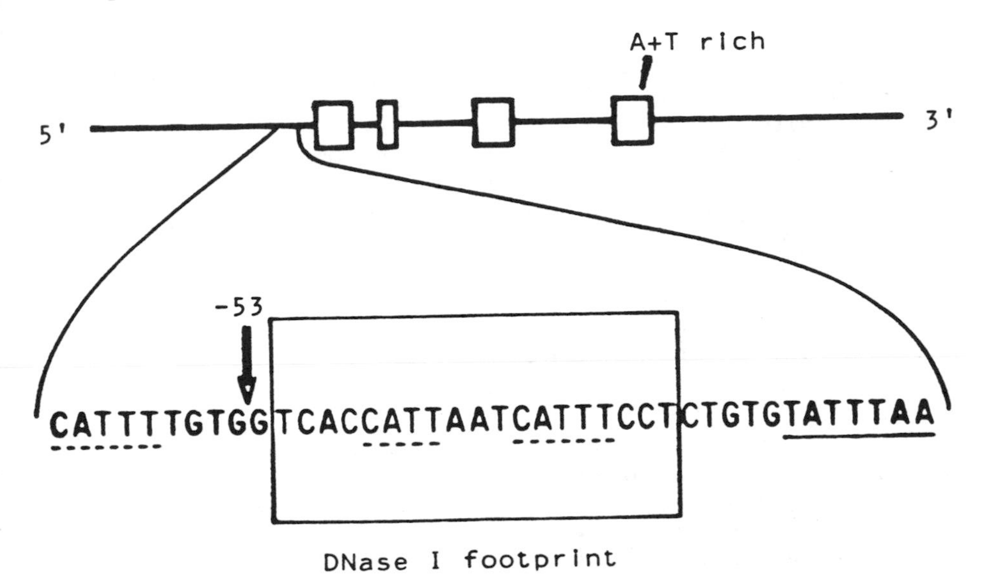

The predominant effects of IL-1 and TNF on GM-CSF messenger RNA accumulation in fibroblasts and endothelial cells are thought to be mediated by stabilization of the messenger RNA; consistent with this observation, these compounds did not enhance expression of recombinant GM-CSF promoter constructs in WI-38 cells. However, treatment of these cells with TPA did result in significant increase in expression of recombinant GM-CSF promoter constructs. Taken together, these results suggest that multiple mechanisms of control are utilized in human fibroblasts to lead to accumulation of GM-CSF messenger RNA and protein. Furthermore, the same promoter sequences shown to be important for GM-CSF expression in lymphocytes are also necessary for constitutive and inducible expression of GM-CSF in fibroblasts (see Figure 3) (Nimer et al., 1989).

SUMMARY

GM-CSF is a potent hematopoietic growth factor which exerts its effects on hematopoietic cell growth both *in vivo* and *in vitro*. In addition, GM-CSF has profound effects enhancing the functional activity of circulating effector cells. GM-CSF can be produced by a variety of cell types in response to immune stimuli; both T-cells and macrophages produce GM-CSF upon activation. Furthermore, activated macrophages secrete IL-1 and TNF, which can stimulate GM-CSF production by certain types of endothelial and fibroblast cells. This local production of GM-CSF could then act on circulating neutrophils, monocytes and eosinophils to enhance their functions in host defense. Thus, one can envision a paracrine system in which the production of GM-CSF is sensitive to immune stimulation, and as a result of GM-CSF production, effector cells are recruited and their activities enhanced (Figure 4). The role of GM-CSF and other CSFs and interleukins in the homeostatic control of hematopoiesis is the subject of intense investigation. Careful integration of molecular and biological studies should yield exciting new information about both the physiologic and therapeutic roles of GM-CSF.

ACKNOWLEDGEMENTS

The authors thank Wendy Aft for careful preparation of the manuscript. The figures are reprinted with permission of the University of California, Riverside-Nichols Institute

Symposium on Cellular and Molecular Endocrinology, 1989.

Figure 4. Role of GM-CSF in Host Defense

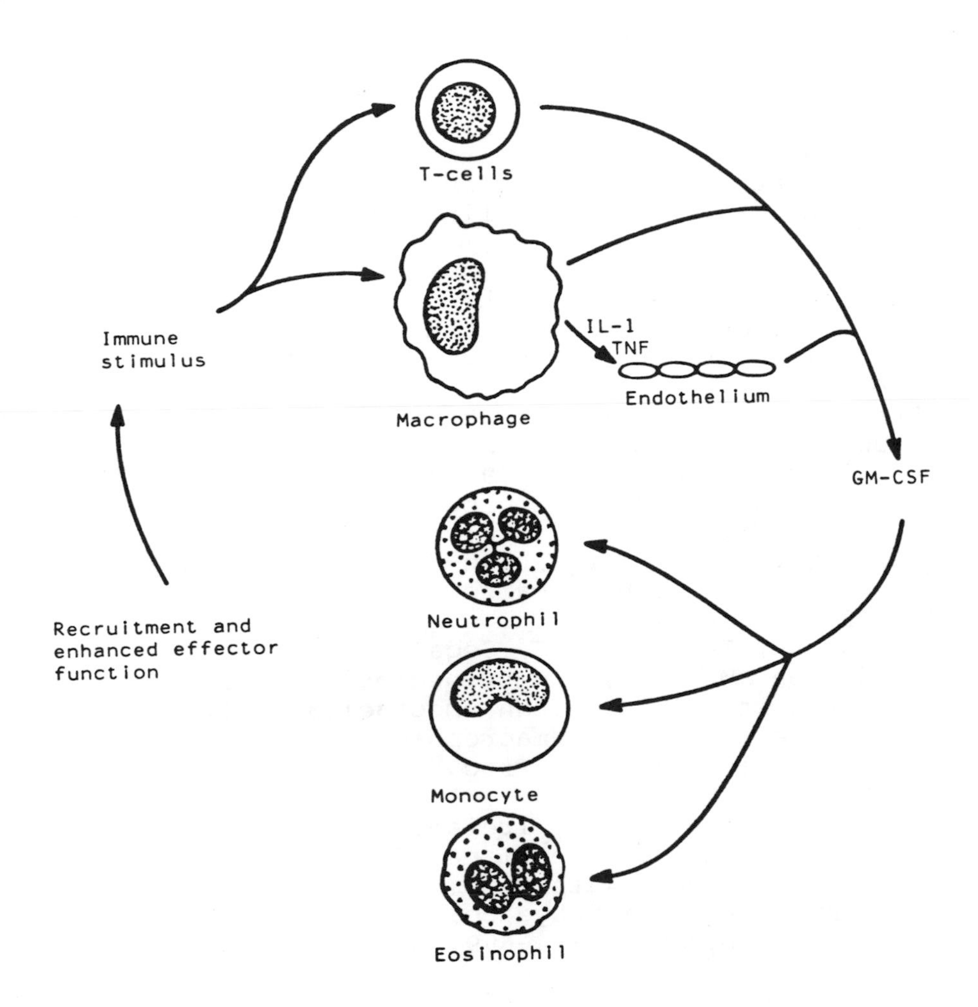

REFERENCES

Antman KS, Griffin JD, Elias A, Socinski MA, Ryan L, Cannistra SA, Oette D, Whitley M, Frei E III, Schnipper LE (1988) Effect of recombinant human granulocyte-macrophage colony-stimulating factor on chemotherapy-induced myelosuppression. New Engl J Med 319:593-598.
Bagby GC, Dinarello CA, Wallace P, Warner C, Hefeneider S, McCall E (1986) Interleukin 1 stimulates granulocyte-macrophage colony-stimulating activity release by vascular endothelial cells. J Clin Invest 78:1316-1323.
Baldwin GC, Gasson JC, Quan SG, Fleischmann J, Weisbart R, Oette D, Mitsuyasu RT, Golde DW (1988) GM-CSF enhances neutrophil function in AIDS patients. Proc Natl Acad Sci USA 85:2763-2766.
Brandt SJ, Peters WP, Atwater SK, Kurtzberg J, Borowitz MJ, Jones RB, Shpall EJ, Bast RC, Gilbert CJ, Oette DH (1988) Effect of recombinant human granulocyte-macrophage colony-stimulating factor on hematopoietic reconstitution after high-dose chemotherapy and autologous bone marrow. New Engl J Med 318:869-876.
Broudy VC, Kaushansky K, Segal GM, Harlan JM, Adamson JW (1986) Tumor necrosis factor type a stimulates human endothelial cells to produce granulocyte/macrophage colony-stimulating factor. Proc Natl Acad Sci USA 83:7467-7471.
Champlin RE, Nimer SD, Ireland P, Oette D, Golde DW (1989) Treatment of refractory aplastic anemia with recombinant human granulocyte-macrophage colony-stimulating factor. Blood 73:694-699.
Chan JY, Slamon DJ, Nimer SD, Golde DW, Gasson JC (1986) Regulation of expression of human granulocyte-macrophage colony-stimulating factor (GM-CSF). Proc Natl Acad Sci USA 83:8669-8673.

Clark SC, Kamen R (1987). The human hematopoietic colony-stimulating factors. Science 236:1229-1236.

DiPersio JF, Billing P, Williams R, Gasson JC (1988) Human granulocyte-macrophage colony-stimulating factor (GM-CSF) and other cytokines prime neutrophils for enhanced arachidonic acid release and leukotriene B_4 synthesis. J Immunol 140:4315-4322.

Golde DW, Gasson JC (1988) Hormones that regulate blood cell production. Scient Am 259:62-70.

Groopman JE, Mitsuyasu RT, DeLeo MJ, Oette DH, Golde DW (1987) Effect of recombinant human granulocyte-macrophage colony-stimulating factor on myelopoiesis in the acquired immunodeficiency syndrome. New Engl J Med 317:593-598.

Huebner K, Isobe M, Croce CM, Golde DW, Kaufman SE, Gasson JC (1985) The human gene encoding GM-CSF is at 5q21-q32, the chromosome region deleted in the 5q- anomaly. Science 230:1282-1285.

Koeffler HP, Gasson J, Tobler A (1988) Transcriptional and posttranscriptional modulation of myeloid colony stimulating factor expression by tumor necrosis factor and other agents. Mol Cell Biol 8:3432-3438.

Le Beau MM, Epstein ND, O'Brien SJ, Nienhuis AW, Yang Y-C, Clark SC, Rowley JD (1987) The interleukin 3 gene is located on human chromosome 5 and is deleted in myeloid leukemias with a deletion of 5q. Proc Natl Acad Sci USA 84:5913-5917.

Le Beau MM, Westbrook CA, Diaz MO, Larson RA, Rowley JD, Gasson JC, Golde DW, Sherr CJ (1986) Evidence for the involvement of GM-CSF and c-fms in the deletion (5q) in myeloid disorders. Science 231:984-987.

Munker R, Gasson J, Ogawa M, Koeffler HP (1986) Recombinant human tumor necrosis factor induces production of granulocyte-monocyte colony-stimulating factor mRNA and protein from lung fibroblasts and vascular

endothelial cells in vitro. Nature 323:79-82.
Naccache PH, Faucher N, Gasson JC, Borgeat P, DiPersio JF (1988) Granulocyte-macrophage colony-stimulating factor modulates the excitation-response coupling sequence in human neutrophils. J Immunol 140:3541-3549.
Nimer SD, Gates MJ, Koeffler HP, Gasson JC (1989) Multiple mechanisms control the expression of GM-CSF by human fibroblasts. J Immunol, in press.
Nimer SD, Morita EA, Martis MJ, Wachsman W, Gasson JC (1988) Characterization of the human granulocyte-macrophage colony-stimulating factor promoter region by genetic analysis: Correlation with DNase I footprinting. Mol Cell Biol 8:1979-1984.
Shaw G, Kamen R (1986) A conserved AU sequence from the 3′ untranslated region of GM-CSF mRNA mediates selective mRNA degradation. Cell 46:659-667.
Silberstein DS, Owen WF, Gasson JC, DiPersio JF, Golde DW, Bina JC, Soberman R, Austen KF, David JR (1986) Regulation of human eosinophil function by granulocyte-macrophage colony-stimulating factor. J Immunol 137:3290-3294.
Tomonaga M, Golde DW, Gasson JC (1986) Biosynthetic (recombinant) human granulocyte-macrophage colony-stimulating factor: effect on normal bone marrow and leukemia cell lines. Blood 67:31-36.
Vadhan-Raj S, Keating M, LeMaistre A, Hittelman WN, McCredie K, Trujillo JM, Broxmeyer HE, Henney C, Gutterman JU (1987) Effects of recombinant human granulocyte-macrophage colony-stimulating factor in patients with myelodysplastic syndromes. New Engl J Med 317:1545-1552.
Weisbart RH, Golde DW, Clark SC, Wong GG, Gasson JC (1985) Human granulocyte-macrophage colony-stimulating factor is a neutrophil activator. Nature 314:361-363.
Weisbart RH, Golde DW, Gasson JC (1986) Biosynthetic human GM-CSF modulates the

number and affinity of neutrophil f-met-leu-phe-receptors. J Immunol 137:3584-3587.

Weisbart RH, Kwan L, Golde DW, Gasson JC (1987) Human GM-CSF primes neutrophils for enhanced oxidative metabolism in response to the major physiologic chemoattractants. Blood 69:18-21.

Wong GG, Witek JS, Temple PA, Wilkens KM, Leary AC, Luxenburg DP, Jones SS, Brown EL, Kay RM, Orr EC, Shoemaker C, Golde DW, Kaufman RJ, Hewick RM, Wang EA, Clark SC (1985) Human GM-CSF: Molecular cloning of the complementary DNA and purification of the natural and recombinant proteins. Science 228:810-815.

Hematopoietic Growth Factors
in Transfusion Medicine, pages 43–63

MACROPHAGE GROWTH AND STIMULATING FACTOR, M-CSF

Peter Ralph and Adam Sampson-Johannes

Department of Cell Biology, Cetus Corporation,
Emeryville, California 94608

INTRODUCTION

Macrophage colony-stimulating factor (M-CSF or CSF-1) is one of a group of proteins that promote the production of blood cells (Clark and Kamen, 1986; Metcalf, 1986; Ralph and Warren, 1988). M-CSF was originally named for its growth promotion of undifferentiated precursors from the bone marrow into colonies of macrophages (Metcalf, 1970; Stanley et al., 1983). However, in addition to *growth* and *differentiation* activities, M-CSF shares with G-CSF and GM-CSF the properties of *maintenance* and *activation* of mature cells (Stanley et al., 1983; Ralph et al., 1986a, 1989).

Bioactivity values of M-CSF in this paper will be that of murine colony forming units measured in mid-titration range (Stanley, 1970; Range et al., 1986b). A different definition is based on 50% of maximum colony formation (Wong et al., 1987), and is about 1/50 of the colony unit that I will use. There is no world standard yet, so units may vary slightly among different labs depending on the mouse strain and culture conditions used.

PRESENCE OF M-CSF IN BODY FLUIDS

M-CSF is one of the few cytokines, intracellular communicating proteins, that is readily detectable in normal human blood, urine, cerebrospinal fluid and fetal amniotic fluid (Table 1). It is present at 2-5 ng/ml in normal human serum and plasma which is 40 pM or 100-300

Table 1. M-CSF in Human Body Fluids

Source		Size (kD) native	Size (kD) SDS	Concentration (ng/ml)	Reference
Normal serum	(n=14)			2.1 ± 0.9[a]	Das et al., 1981
	(n-10)			2.3 ± 0.2[b]	Shadle et al., 1989
term gravid	(n=6)			3.4	Ringler et al., 1988
cord	(n=6)			3.0	Ringler et al., 1988
Normal plasma	(n=10)		48(-140)	2.4 ± 0.3[b]	Shadle et al., 1989
Adult urine	(pool)		82	10[a]	Sakai et al., 1987
	(pool)		57	9[a]	Tao et al., 1987
		85	46		Wang & Goldwasser, 1983
			80		Wong et al., 1987
selected geriatric		45-90	45	7-18[a]	Das et al., 1981
Amniotic fluid					
term	(n=11)			4.6	Ringler et al., 1988
mid-trimester	(n=20)			5.1 ± 0.5	Cox et al., unpublished
term; normal, induced or no labor	(n=37)			11.1 ± 1.9	Cox et al., unpublished
Cerebrospinal fluid	(n=19)		0.6 ± 0.1		Ralph & Frei, unpublished
Arthritis joint fluid	(n=1)		12		Firestein et al., 1988

[a]based on purified urinary 45 kd M-CSF, S.A. ~5x10^7 U/mg, I U = 12 pg

[b]based on purified, bacterial 45 kd (SDS) rM-CSF with 150 amino acid monomers. S.A. ~ 1.4x10^8 U/mg, 1 U = 20 pg

U/ml (Das et al., 1981; Shadle et al., 1989). This is at the threshold for biological effects (see below).

M-CSF levels are elevated in infection or inflammatory conditions. High titers of M-CSF are seen in serum, cerebrospinal fluid, and amniotic fluid during bacterial infections or after severe burns (Table 2). Injection of endotoxin, tumor necrosis factor (TNF) (Table 2) or IL-2 (Fibbe, unpublished) into cancer patients also raises M-CSF concentrations. Sera of cancer patients often have elevated M-CSF levels, e.g. in mammary and ovarian carcinoma but not in hairy cell leukemia (Table 2).

Levels of M-CSF in body fluids of mice are considerably higher than reported in humans. Serum levels rise from 1000 U/ml to 32,000 U/ml during lethal *Listeria monocytogenes* infections (Cheers et al., 1988).

During pregnancy there is a 10,000-fold increase in M-CSF protein in the mouse uterus which is hormonally regulated. In situ hybridization shows that expression is localized to the luminal and glandular secretory epithelial cells of the endometrium at the sites of implantation of the developing blastocyst (Pollard et al., 1987). The juxtaposing trophoblasts of the growing placenta are the only cell type other than macrophage-related cells to express M-CSF receptors. M-CSF levels are found in murine amniotic fluid at up to 10 times the normal adult serum levels (Azoulay et al., 1987). This suggests that M-CSF is involved in the growth and maintenance of the placenta during pregnancy.

STRUCTURE OF THE M-CSF GENE, ITS TRANSCRIPTS, AND PROTEIN

M-CSF is considerable more complex in genetic and protein structure than other hemopoietic factors, IL-1 through IL-7, G-CSF, and GM-CSF. M-CSF is the only dimer, of molecular weight ranging from 45 to 100 kd depending on both carbohydrate and amino acid differences (Wong et al., 1987; Ladner et al., 1987; Shadle et al., 1987). Cloning of several human cDNA's, sequencing of the gene, and amino acid sequencing show the following structures (Table 3). The gene is about 21 kb in length, and has 10 possible exons. It can generate at least 7 sizes of cytoplasmic mRNA from 1.6 to 4.5 kb using alternately splicing sites in exon 6, or whole alternate exons for 3' untranslated regions (Ladner et al., 1987). M-CSF mRNA is found in a number of murine (Rajavashisth et al., 1987;

Table 2. Condition of Altered M-CSF Levels

Infection/Inflammation		Concentration ng/ml	Reference
Burn patient sera, septic	(n=20)	20 ± 1[a]	Peterson et al., 1988
non-septic	(n=20)	14 ± 2	
Burn patient urine	(n=5)	(10-80)[b]	Sampson-Johannes & Peterson, unpublished
Post-TNF serum	(n=5)	45 ± 13[c]	Sampson-Johannes & Spriggs, unpublished
Cerebrospinal fluid			Ralph & Frei, unpublished
normal	(n=19)[d]	0.6 ± 0.1	
bacterial infection	(n=9)	21.0 ± 4.9	
viral infection	(n=5)	1.8 ± 0.3	
brain tumor	(n=8)	2.3 ± 0.5	
Amniotic fluid, pre-term			Cox et al., unpublished
normal	(n=5)	14.3 ± 5.7	
endotoxin-positive	(n=7)	36.1 ± 8.8	
<u>Cancer</u>			
Ovarian, plasma			Kacinski et al., 1989
without active disease	(n=63)	3.8 ± 0.2(0-6.7)[e]	
active or recurrent disease	(n=41)	11.6 ± 1.5(1.1-40)	
Ovarian	(n=14)	11.1 ± 1.1[f]	
Mammary	(n=27)	8.8 ± 1.0[f]	Ralph & Kufe, unpublished
Hairy cell leukemia	(n=21)	5.2 ± 0.1[g]	Ralph & Fibbe, unpublished

[a] At peak 7-14 days post-burn
[b] Range of maxima occurring 10-30 days post-burn
[c] At 24-hour peak, the last time point assayed
[d] Includes normal (n=5), multiple sclerosis (n=9), other neurological diseases (n=5)
[e] Range
[f] Normals from the same hospital = 5.3 ± 0.3 ng/ml (n=30)
[g] Normals from the same hospital = 5.8 ± 0.2 ng/ml (n=7)

Table 3. Human M-CSF Molecular Structure

Gene		10 exons	21 kb	Ladner et al., 1987
mRNA	Size (kb)	Exon 6 usage (base number)	Propolypeptide (aa)	Reference
α	1.6	764-894	224	Kawasaki et al., 1985
β	~4.0	1-894	522	Wong et al., 1987
				Ladner et al., 1987
γ		253-894	438	Cerretti et al., 1988
δ		1-573	340	Otsuka, 1987

Circulating Protein Hormone

Form	mRNA used	Monomer (aa)	Apparent size (kd) native	Apparent size (kd) SDS
short	α	153-158	48-65	40-43
long	β (γ, δ)	~223	70-100	

Pollard et al., 1987; Azoulay et al., 1987; Troutt and Lee, 1989) and human tissues (Wong et al., 1987; Wang et al., unpublished), and is predominately of the largest 4.0-4.5 kb size.

cDNA cloning has defined 4 species of human mRNA for M-CSF, named α to δ, which specify 4 different primary polypeptides (Table 3). The shortest polypeptide α contains a precursor of 224 amino acids plus an N-terminal 32 amino acid signal sequence (Kawasaki et al., 1985). The longest cDNA, β, specifies a precursor of 522 amino acids plus the same 32 residue leader (Wong et al., 1987; Ladner et al., 1987). The two polypeptide sequences are the same except that the long one has an additional 298 amino acids inserted after the common residue at position 149. The amino acid numbering will refer to residues in the propolypeptide not counting the leader sequence. The γ molecule also specifies an insert after position 149, but of only the first 214 additional residues of β (Cerretti et al., 1988). The α, β and γ polypeptides all end with a 23 residue hydrophobic region followed by 36 residues of a "cytoplasmic" tail. The hydrophobic region and subsequent "anchor" of 4 basic amino acids are encoded by a separate exon (Ladner et al., 1987) and are typical of a transmembrane protein (Kawasaki et al., 1985). α, β, and γ cDNA's were obtained from a pancreatic carcinoma cell line MIA PaCa. β was also derived from an SV40-transformed trophoblast cell line TPA30-1 and a clone of the T cell line CEM. The δ cDNA from CEM specifies a polypeptide which continues past residue 149 as β and γ, but apparently ends at position 340 and lacks the C-terminal transmembrane and cytoplastic tail structure (Otsuka, 1987).

Cellular processing results in extensive deletions of C-terminal regions, so that basically two kinds of dimer molecules are secreted, a short form of 153-158 amino acid monomers (Rettenmier et al., 1987; Halenbeck et al., 1988) and a long form of about 223 amino acid monomers (Wong et al., 1987; Halenbeck et al., 1989). M-CSF can be further truncated at the C-terminus to end at residue 150 while retaining full biological activity (Halenbeck et al., 1989 and unpublished). Molecules genetically engineered to end at 147 (Otsuka, 1987) and 149 (Arretti et al., 1988) are also reported to be bioactive. The human T cell line appears to process a further 2 or 4 amino acids at the N-terminus of M-CSF without loss of bioactivity (Takahashi et al., 1988).

GENETIC LOCATION AND EVOLUTIONARY CONSIDERATIONS

The human M-CSF gene is located on the long arm of chromosome 5 at 5q33.1 (Pettenati et al., 1987), very close to the gene for its receptor, the proto-oncogene *c-fms* (Sherr et al., 1985) at 5q33.2-3 (Roberts et al., 1988). There seems to be a reason for the close association because I am unaware of any other vertebrate ligand gene and its receptor gene being anywhere on the same chromosome. The platelet-derived growth factor (PDGF) receptor gene is highly homologous to *c-fms* and is immediately adjacent to it (Roberts et al., 1988). PDGF is a dimer like M-CSF. The similarities of the two receptor-ligand systems are intriguing but there is no apparent amino acid or nucleic homology between M-CSF and PDGF. Other hemopoietic growth factor genes are also on the long arm of chromosome 5: GM-CSF, IL3, IL4 and IL5 (Sutherland et al., 1988) (Fig. 1). This association appears to be fortuitous since in the mouse the M-CSF gene has been located to chromosome 3 (Gisselbrecht et al., 1989), whereas GM-CSF, IL3, IL4 and IL5 are on chromosome 11 (Lee et al., 1989a) and the M-CSF-R gene is on chromosome 18 (Wang et al., 1988).

Recombinant proteins containing only the first 150 amino acids of M-CSF are active, so why does the gene code for 522 amino acids with a C-terminus like an integral transmembrane protein? Comparison of the long human γ cDNA with homologous murine cDNA's (DeLamarter et al., 1987; Ladner et al., 1988) shows that the amino acid residues are 81% identical over the minimum active length around 150 amino acids. There is also an 81% identity over the next 73 residues which are present in the predominant long form of the natural protein but are not necessary for full biological activity. The remaining regions, perimembrane, transmembrane and cytoplasmic, are 56-87% identical (Ralph et al., 1989). All 9 cysteines are conserved between human and mouse, yet the last two at positions 159 and 161 can be mutated to alanine or serine without loss of activity (Koths et al., unpublished). This suggests that the complete membrane-associated polypeptide has evolved for an unknown role different from that of the released hormone. A similar puzzle is seen with the family of epidermal growth factor/transforming growth factor proteins in which the secreted hormone is a small part of a polypeptide with integral membrane properties (Ralph et al., 1987). There is some unpublished evidence for a surface membrane form of M-CSF, which is released slowly from producing cells

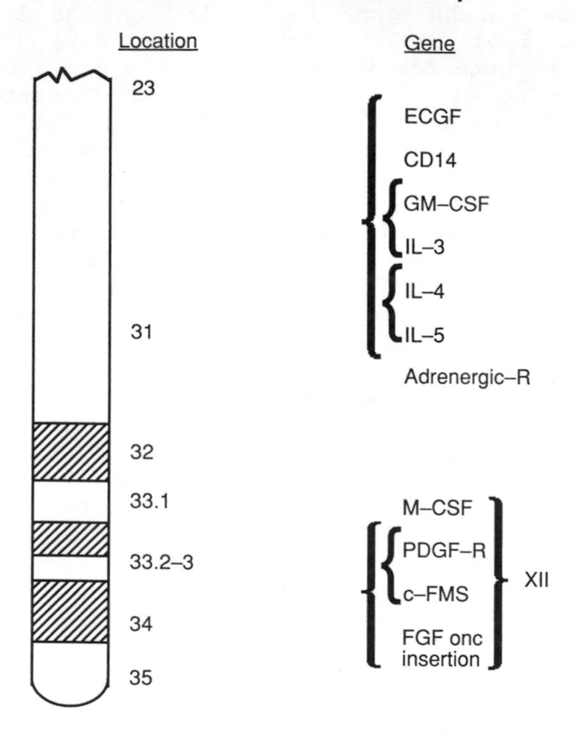

Figure 1. Location of M-CSF on human chromosome 5. See text and Ralph et al., 1989 for a description of the other genes shown.

as a soluble fragment (Rettenmier et al., 1987), being active as a macrophage growth factor.

NORMAL CELL PRODUCTION OF M-CSF

Several cell types produce M-CSF constitutively *ex vivo*, including fibroblasts, endothelial cells and epithelial cells (Ralph 1989, Ralph et al., 1989; Lee et al., 1988). Induction of these cells with LPS, pIC, or IL1 that increases GM-CSF and G-CSF production has little effect of the continued secretion of M-CSF (Fibbe et al., 1988, 1989). M-CSF is not detected in mitogen-induced human blood cell or murine spleen cell conditioned medium (Ralph and Nakoinz 1987; Nakoinz and Ralph, 1988) which are rich in lymphokines.

Human monocytes are capable of producing M-CSF for their own use. Simple adherence induces high levels of mRNA, but endotoxin (Haskill et al., 1988; Lee et al., 1989b) or other second signal (Vellenga et al., 1988) is required for efficient production of the hormone. Induction of M-CSF gene expression is apparently tightly regulated by autonomous prostaglandin production. PEG2 preferentially inhibits induction of M-CSF transcripts compared to G-CSF or GM-CSF transcripts in adherent monocytes, and indomethacin, an inhibitor of PGE production, greatly stimulates induction of transcripts and secretion of the protein (Lee at al., 1989b).

BIOLOGICAL ACTIVITY OF DIFFERENT FORMS OF HUMAN AND MURINE M-CSF

Growth Factor

M-CSF induces the formation of granulocyte colonies from mouse bone marrow cells within a few days in semi-solid culture, and predominantly macrophage colonies at later times (Metcalf, 1970). M-CSF also induces the liquid culture growth of murine macrophages from marrow precursors, although better results are obtained with L-cell conditioned medium, a crude source of M-CSF plus other undefined co-factors (Stanley, 1985).

Human M-CSF has a specific activity similar to the murine protein in a murine bone marrow colony-forming assay, about 10^8 U/mg, but murine M-CSF is inactive on human cells. Plateau levels occur at 100-200 U/ml and half maximum colony formation titrates at about 50 U/ml. M-CSF induces liquid or semi-solid growth of macrophages from cultures of murine peritoneal and long macrophages and blood monocytes (reviewed by Chen et al., 1988).

We adapted an IL3-dependent murine myeloid cell line NFS-60 to growth with M-CSF as a convenient bioassay (Nakoinz et al., 1989). Human and murine M-CSF have similar specific activities in this assay.

Human M-CSF produces colonies, generally of less than 50 cells, from human bone marrow. The colonies are composed of disperse, large esterase-positive macrophages (Das et al., 1981; Ralph et al., 1986b; Motoyoshi et al.,

1989). The response of donor marrow cells varies greatly in comparison to the mouse, and fewer colonies are formed per 10^5 cells cultured. We find that M-CSF exhibits a plateau in this assay at 10^3-10^4 U/ml and a half maximum at about 500 U/ml (Ralph et al., 1986b).

A series of experiments on human M-CSF short form of 150-158 amino acid monomers, and long form of about 220 amino acid monomers, showed no difference by these in vitro growth assays. Proteins were purified to >95% from human urine (Kawasaki et al., 1985) or human MIA PaCa cells (Boosman et al., 1987), or after recombinant production in monkey (Halenbeck et al., 1988), insect, or bacterial cells (Halenbeck et al., 1989). High level production from *E. coli* required recombinant engineering for over-expression of suitable monomer species and careful biochemical manipulation to achieve the proper disulfide bonds and final molecular configuration (Halenbeck et al., 1989).

Maintenance

M-CSF maintains the viability and biochemical functions of populations of murine peritoneal and bone marrow-derived macrophages, and of factor-dependent macrophage lines (Tushinshi et al., 1982; Morgan et al., 1987). Human M-CSF greatly improves the survival of human monocytes for weeks in serum-free cultures and in some conditions in human serum (Becker et al., 1987; Gundlemann et al., 1988). Low levels of DNA synthesis (thymidine incorporation) (Kufe et al., 1988; Gundlemann et al., 1988), mitotic indices (Gundlemann et al., 1988) and cell growth (Sechler et al., 1989) are found in M-CSF treated monocyte cultures.

Stimulation Factor for Mature Cells

M-CSF *in vitro* stimulates a number of functions of monocytes and macrophages, including production of cytokines, enzymes, prostaglandins, and reactive oxygen intermediates (Table 4). It stimulates nonspecific and antibody-dependent cellular cytotoxicity (ADCC), killing of *Candida* and *Mycobacterium avium*, resistance to viral infection, and suppression of T cell response. On the other hand, M-CSF as well as IL3 and GM-CSF enhances the replication of human immunodeficiency virus (HIV) in monocytes (Gendleman et al., 1988; Koyanagi et al., 1988;

Table 4. M-CSF is a Stimulating Factor for Mature Monocytes and Macrophages

Function	References	
	Human Monocyte	Murine Macrophage
Production of G-CSF		*
Production of IFN, TNF and myeloid CSF	Warren & Ralph, 1986	*
Production of prostaglandin E, plasminogen activator, ferritin, IL-1, peroxide		*
Production of procoagulant	Lyberg et al., 1987	Lyberg et al., 1987
Formation of osteoclast-like cells	Van deWijngaert, 1987	#
Tumoricidal activity	Sampson-Johannes & Carlino, 1988	Ralph & Nakoinz, 1987
Antibody-dependent tumorilysis	Munn & Cheung, 1988	Nakoinz & Ralph, 1988
Killing of MAI (*Mycobacterium avium*)	Bermudez & Young, 1989	Bermudez & Young, 1989
Survival, acid phosphatase, surface antigens	Becker et al., 1987	
Replication of HIV (AIDS virus) together with GM-CSF	Gendleman et al., 1988	
Inhibition of vesicular stomatitis virus		Lee & Warren, 1987
Intracellular killing of *Candida*		Karbassi et al., 1987

* Reviewed by Ralph et al., 1986a
# M-CSF inhibited osteoclast-like cell proliferation in mouse bone marrow culture (MacDonald et al., 1986)

Perno et al., 1989). Approximately 1000 U/ml is optimal for almost all of these effects, as it is for colony formation by human bone marrow, but in contrast to 100 U/ml required for murine bone marrow colonies.

M-CSF AND LEUKEMOGENESIS

A fraction of fresh human myeloid leukemic cell samples of several types express M-CSF mRNA or secrete the protein, and a partially overlapping subset expresses M-CSF receptors (Rambaldi et al., 1988). Thus, an autocrine proliferation via M-CSF may have a role in the leukemogenesis or progression of some myeloid cancers. The human *c-fms* receptor gene is not oncogenic alone, but when expressed together with its normal ligand, M-CSF transforms mouse 3T3 into tumorigenic cells (Roussell et al., 1986).

No CSF or CSF receptor has been identified in humans in an oncogene state (gross overproduction or altered, permanently signaling receptor). Expression of M-CSF in acute myeloblastic leukemia (AML) cells is correlated with poor growth in culture (Miyauchi et al., 1988). G-, GM-, or multi-CSF (IL-3) often stimulates growth of AML in culture, and in 75% of cases addition of M-CSF inhibits growth and induces differentiation to nondividing macrophages (Miyauchi et al., 1988). It may therefore be preferable to use M-CSF instead of the other CSFs in clinical trails in myeloid leukemia and preleukemia to restore normal blood granulocyte and monocyte levels.

PRECLINICAL STUDIES IN EXPERIMENTAL ANIMALS

Pharmacologic doses of murine and recombinant human M-CSF increase blood granulocyte and monocyte levels, tissue macrophage numbers, cycling of marrow progenitors and greatly increase the splenic content of progenitors (Table 5). The stimulatory effects of M-CSF on precursors for granulocytes, megakaryocytes and erythrocytes (Broxmeyer et al., 1987) is presumably due to an indirect action *in vivo*. M-CSF stimulates NK activity, macrophage and monocyte ADCC, protects against lethal *E. coli* and candida infection in normal and cytoxan-suppressed mice, and reduces tumor metastases and increases survival in mouse B16 melanoma model. It synergizes with IFN and local irradiation in the treatment of mice with B16 and Lewis lung carcinoma tumors.

Table 5. Preclinical Efficacy Studies of M-CSF

Study	Reference
Mouse	
Increase tissue macrophages	Lotem & Sachs, 1988
	Ralph et al., 1989
Increase blood monocytes and granulocytes	Chong & Langlois, 1988
	Hume, 1988
Extramedullary hematopoiesis	Broxmeyer et al., 1987
	Ralph et al., 1989
Stimulate spleen NK activity	Chong et al., 1989
Stimulate peritoneal macrophage ADCC	Ralph et al., 1989
Reduce B16 melanoma metastases, increase survival	Hume,1989
	Young et al., 1989
Cancer treatment synergy with IFNγ and X-rays	Lu et al., 1989
Protect against lethal *E. coli* infection	Chong & Langlois, 1988
Protect against lethal *Candida albicans* infection	Chong & Langlois, 1989
Block myelosuppression caused by interferons	Koren et al., 1986
Monkey	
Cynomolgus: Increase monocyte numbers and ADCC	Munn & Cheung, 1988
	Donahue et al., 1988
Rhesus: Increase monocyte numbers	Nachtman, unpublished
Rabbit	
Increase blood monocytes	Garnick, 1989

Toxicity studies show mainly thrombocytopenia with moderate anemia in rodents and primates (Nachtman, unpublished; Garnick, 1989), apparently due to consumption by macrophages. Lowered cholesterol levels were seen in rabbits and cynomolgus monkeys treated with high doses of M-CSF, near a milligram/Kg/day (Garnick, 1989). Similar cholesterol lowering was reported for administration of GM-CSF to aplastic anemia patients (Nimer et al., 1988).

CLINICAL TRIALS

Clinical trials have been in progress in Japan for several years using partially purified urinary M-CSF. Results show enhanced serum G-CSF activity and monocyte production of G-CSF ex vivo (Ishizaka et al., 1986), increased blood neutrophil levels in cancer patients who are myelosuppressed by their chemotherapy (Matsumoto et al., 1987), and increased blood neutrophils in chronic neutropenia of childhood (Komiyama et al., 1988), and increased leukocyte recovery after bone marrow transplantation (Masaoka et al., 1988).

Cetus Corporation and Genetics Institute have just started clinical trials in cancer patients using recombinant M-CSF.

ACKNOWLEDGMENTS

We thank the Cetus Assay Lab for M-CSF determinations and D. Jackson and K. Levenson for expert editorial assistance.

REFERENCES

Azoulay M, Webb CG, Sachs L (1987) Control of hematopoietic cell growth regulators during mouse fetal development. Mol Cell Biol 7:3361-3364.

Bartocci A, Pollard JW, Stanley ER (1986) Regulation of colony-stimulating factor 1 during pregnancy. J Exp Med 164:956-961.

Becker SJ, Devlin RB, Haskill JS (1988) Differential production of tumor necrosis factor (TNF), macrophage colony stimulating factor (CSF1) and interleukin-1 (IL1) by human alveolar macrophages. J Leuk Biol 45:353-361.

Bermudez LE, Young LS (1989) Presented at Amer Soc Clin Invest.

Boosman A, Strickler J, Wilson K (1987) Partial primary structures of human and murine macrophage colony stimulating factor (CSF-1). Biochem Biophys Res 144:74-80.

Broxmeyer HE, Williams DE, Hangoc G (1987) Synergistic actions in vivo after administration to mice of combinations of purified natural murine colony-stimulating factor 1, recombinant interleukin-2 and recombinant granulocyte-macrophage colony stimulating factor. Proc Natl Acad Sci USA 84:3871-3875.

Cerretti DP, Wignall J, Anderson D (1988) Human macrophage colony stimulating factor: alternative RNA and protein processing from a single gene. Mol Immunol 25:761-770.

Cheers C, Haigh AM, Kelso A, Metcalf D, Stanley ER, Young AM (1988) Production of colony-stimulating factors (CSFs) during infection: separate determinations of macrophage-, granulocyte-, granulocyte-macrophage-, and multi-CSFs. Infect Immun 56:247-251.

Chen BD-M, Mueller M, Chou T-H (1988) Role of granulocyte/ macrophage colony-stimulating factor in the regulation of murine alveolar macrophage proliferation and differentiation. (1988) J Immunol 141:139-144.

Chong KT, Langlois L (1988) Enhancing effect of macrophage colony-stimulating factor (MCSF) on leukocytes and host defense in normal and immunosuppressed mice. FASEB J 2:A1474.

Chong KT, Langlois L (1989) Recombinant human macrophage colony-stimulating factor (M-CSF) stimulates mouse resistance to lethal *Candida albicans* infections. Presented at Am Soc Microbiol.

Chong KT, Langlois L, Doyle (1989) Recombinant human macrophage colony-stimulating factor (M-CSF) enhanced murine splenic natural-killer (NK) cell activity. FASEB J 3:A816.

Clark SC, Kamen R (1987) The human hematopoietic colony-stimulating factors. Science 236:1229-1237.

Das SK, Stanley ER, Guilbert LJ, Forman LW (1981) Human colony-stimulating factor (CSF-1) radioimmunoassay: resolution of three subclasses of human colony-stimulating factors. Blood 58:630.

DeLamarter JF, Hession C, Semon (1987) Nucleotide sequence of a cDNA encoding murine CSF-1 (macrophage-CSF). Nucl Acids Res 15:2389-2390.

Donahue RE, Wong GG, Metzger M, Seghal PK, Morris JP, Turner KJ, Morin SH, Sibley SB, Stoudemire J, Clark SC, Garnick M (1988) In vivo effects of recombinant human macrophage-colony stimulating factor (M-CSF) in primates. Blood 72(S1):114a.

Fibbe WE, van Damme J (1988) Human fibroblasts produce G-, M- and GM-CSF following stimulation by IL-1 and poly IC. Blood 72:860-866.

Fibbe WE, Daha M (1989) IL-1 and poly IC induce production of G-, M-, GM-CSF by human endothelial cells. Exp Hematol 17:229-234.

Firestein GS, Xu W-D, Townsend K, Broide D, Alvaro-Gracia J, Glasebroo A, Zvaifler NJ (1988) Cytokines in chronic inflammatory arthritis. J Exp Med 168:1573.

Garnick M (1989) Presented at Workshop on Regulatory Issues for Hematopoietic Growth Factors. Bethesda, MD.

Gendleman H, Orenstein JM, Martin MA (1988) Efficient isolation and propagation of human immunodeficiency virus on recombinant colony-stimulating factor 1-treated monocytes. J Exp Med 167:1428-1441.

Gilbert HS, Praloran V, Stanley ER (1989) Increased circulating CSF-1 (M-CSF) in myeloproliferative disease: association with myeloid metaplasia and peripheral bone marrow extension. Blood, in press.

Gisselbrecht S, Sola B, Fichelson S, Bordereaux D, Tambourin P (1989) The murine M-CSF gene is localized on chromsome 3. Blood 73:1742-1745.

Halenbeck R, Shadle P, Lee P-J, Lee MT, Koths K (1988) Purification and characterization of recombinant human macrophage colony stimulating factor and generation of a neutralizing antibody useful for Western analysis. J Biotech 8:45-58.

Halenbeck R, Kawasaki E, Wrin J, Koths K (1989) Renaturation and purification of recombinant human macrophage colony-stimulating factor expressed in *E. coli*. BioTech, in press.

Haskill S, Johnson C, Eierman D (1988) Adherence induced selective mRNA expression of monocyte mediators and proto-oncogenes. J Immunol 140:1690-1694.

Hume DA, Pavli P, Donahue RE, Fidler IJ (1988) The effect of human recombinant macrophage colony-stimulating factor (CSF-1) on the murine mononuclear phagocyte system *in vivo*. J Immunol 141:3405-3409.

Hume D, Donahue RE, Fidler IJ (1989) The therapeutic effect of human recombinant macrophage colony stimulating factor (CSF-1) in experimental murine metastatic melanoma. Lymphokine Res 32:127.

Ishizaka Y, Motoyoshi K, Hatake K (1986) Mode of action of human urinary colony-stimulating factor. Exp Hematol 14:1-8.

Kacinski BM, Stanley ER, Carter D, Chamgers JT, Chambers SK, Kohorn EI, Schwartz PE (1989) Circulating levels of CSF-1 (M-CSF) a lymphohematopoietic cytokine may be a useful marker of disease status in patients with malignant ovarian neoplasms. Int J Radiation Oncology Biol Phys 17, in press.

Karbassi A, Becker JM, Foster JS (1987) Enhanced killing of *Candida albicans* by murine macrophages treated with macrophage colony-stimulating factor: evidence for augmented expression of mannose receptors. J Immunol 139:417-421.

Kaushansky K, Broudey VC, Harlan JM, Adamson JW (1988) Tumor necrosis factor-alpha and tumor necrosis factor-beta (lymphotoxin) stimulate the production of granulocyte-macrophage colony-stimulating factor, macrophage colony-stimulating factor, and IL-1 *in vivo*. J Immunol 141:3410-3415.

Kawasaki ES, Ladner MB, Wang AM (1985) Molecular cloning of a complementary DNA encoding human macrophage-specific colony-stimulating factor (CSF-1). Science 230:291-296.

Komiyama A (1988) Increases in neutrophil counts by purified human urinary colony-stimulating factor in chronic neutropenia of childhood. Blood 71:41-45.

Koren S, Klimpel GR, Fleischmann WR (1986) Macrophage colony stimulating factor (CSF-1) blocks the myeloid suppressive but not the antiviral or antiproliferative activities of murine alpha, beta, and gamma interferons *in vitro*. J Biol Response Modif 5:571-580.

Koyanagi Y, O'Brien WA, Zhao JQ, Golde DW, Gasson JC, Chen ISY (1988) Cytokines alter production of HIV-1 from primary mononuclear phagocytes. Science 241:1673.

Ladner MB, Martin GA, Noble JA (1987) Human CSF-1: gene structure and alternative splicing of mRNA precursors. EMBO J 6:2693-2698.

Ladner MB, Martin GA, Noble JA (1988) cDNA cloning and expression of murine CSF-1 from L929 cells. Proc Natl Acad Sci USA 85:6706-6710.

Le PT, Kurtzber J, Brandt SJ, Niedel JE, Haynes BF, Singer KH (1988) Human thymic epithelial cells produce granulocyte and macrophage colony-stimulating factors. J Immunol 141:1211-1217.

Lee JS, Campbell HD, Kozak CA, Yound IG (1989) IL-4 and IL-5 genes are closely linked and are part of a cytokine gene cluster on mouse chromosome II. Somat Cell Molec Genet 15:2.

Lee MT, Kaushausky K, Ralph P, Ladner MD (1989) Differential expression of M-CSF, G-CSF and GM-CSF by human monocytes. J Leuk Biol, in press.

Lotem J, Sachs L (1988) In vivo control of differentiation of myeloid leukemic cells by rGM-CSF and IL-3. Blood 71:375-382.

Lu L, Shen RN, Lin ZH, Aukerman SL, Broxmeyer HE (1989) Antitumor effects of recombinant cytokines (IL-1α, IL-6, CSF-1, IFN-γ), alone or in combination with local irradiation, in mice inoculated with Lewis lung carcinoma cells. Exp Hematol 17:581.

Lyberg T, Stanley ER, Prydz H (1987) Colony-stimulating factor-1 induces thromboplastin activity in murine macrophages and human monocytes. J Cell Physiol 132:367-376.

MacDonald BR, Mundy GR, Clark S (1986) Effects of human recombinant CSF-GM and highly purified CSF-1 on the formation of multinucleated cells with osteoclast characteristics in long-term bone marrow cultures. J Bone Miner Res 1:227-233.

Masaoka T, Motoyoshi K, Takaku F, Kato S, Harada M, Kodera Y, Kanamaru A, Moriyama Y, Ohno R, Ohira M, Shibata H, Inoue T (1988) Administration of human urinary colony stimulating factor after bone marrow transplantation. Bone Marrow Transplantation 3:121-127.

Matsumoto K, Kakizoe T, Nakagami Y (1987) Clinical trial of CSF-HU (colony-stimulating factor derived from human urine: P-100) on granulocytopenia induced by anticancer therapy in urogenital cancer patients. Hinyokikia Kiyo (Japan) 33:972-982.

Metcalf D (1970) Studies on colony formation in vitro by mouse bone marrow cells. J Cell Physiol 76:89-100.

Metcalf D (1986) The molecular biology and functions of the GM-CSF. Blood 67:257-267.

Miyauchi J, Minden MD, McCulloch EA (1987) The effect of recombinant human CSF-1 on acute myeloblastic leukemia (AML) cells in culture. Blood 70(1):264a.

Morgan C, Pollard JW, Stanley ER (1987) Isolation and characterization of a cloned growth factor dependent macrophage cell line, BAC1.2F5. J Cellular Physiology 130:420-427.

Motoyoshi K, Yoshida K, Hatake K (1989) Recombinant and native human urinary colony-stimulating factor directly augments granulocytic and granulocyte-macrophage colony-stimulating factor production of human peripheral blood monocytes. Exp Hematol 17:68-71.

Munn DH, Cheung N-KY (1988) Recombinant macrophage colony-stimulating factor (M-CSF) induced high levels of anti-tumor antibody-dependent cellular cytotoxicity (ADCC) by cultured human monocytes. Blood 72(1):127a.

Nakoinz I, Ralph P (1988) Stimulation of macrophage ADCC to tumor targets by lymphokines and rCSF-1. Cell Immunol 116:331-340.

Nakoinz I, Lee MT, Weaver JF, Ralph P (1989) Differentiation of the IL-3-dependent NFS-60 cell line and adaption to growth in M-CSF, submitted.

Nimer SD, Champlin RE, Golde DW (1988) Serum cholesterol-lowering activity of granulocyte-macrophage colony-stimulating factor. JAMA 260:3297.

Otsuka European Patent Application. 0 261 592, filed September 17, 1987.

Perno C-F, Yarchoan R, Cooney DA, Hartman NR, Webb DSA, Hao Z, Mitsuya H, Johns DG, Broder S (1989) Replication of human immunodeficiency virus in monocytes. J Exp Med 169:933-951.

Peterson V, Ralph P, Kaushansky K, Sampson-Johannes A, Rundus, C (1988) Impact of sepsis on the macrophage-colony stimulating factor (M-CSF) response to inflammation following thermal injury. Blood 72:131a.

Pattenati MJ, LeBeau MM, Lemons RS (1987) Assignment of CSF-1 to 5q33.1: evidence for clustering of genes regulating haematopoiesis and for their involvement in the deletion of the long arm of chromosome 5 in myeloid disorders. Proc Natl Acad Sci USA 84:2970-2974.

Pollard JW, Bartocci A, Arceci R. (1987) Apparent role of the macrophage growth factor, CSF-1, in placental development. Nature 330:484-486.

Rajavashisth TB, Eng R, Shadduck RK (1987) Cloning and tissue-specific expression of mouse macrophage colony-stimulating factor mRNA. Proc Natl Acad Sci USA 84:1157-1161.

Ralph P (1989) Colony stimulating factors. In Asherson L, Zambala M (eds): "Human Monocytes," New York: Academic Press, in press.

Ralph P, Nakoinz I (1987) Stimulation of macrophage tumoricidal activity by CSF-1. Cell Immunol 105:270-279.

Ralph P, Warren MK (1988) Molecular biology, cell biology and clinical future of myeloid growth factors. In Cruse JM, Lewis RE (eds): "The Year in Immunology 1988; Immunoregulatory Cytokines and Cell Growth," Karger S, Basel AG, pp 103-125.

Ralph P, Warren MK, Ladner MB (1986a) Molecular and biological properties of human CSF-1. Cold Spring Harbor Symp Quant Biol 51:679-683.

Ralph P, Warren MK, Lee MT (1986b) Inducible production of human macrophage growth factor, CSF-1. Blood 68:633-639.

Ralph P, Ladner MB, Wang AM (1987) The molecular and biological properties of the human and murine members of the CSF-1 family. In Webb DR, Pierce CS, Cohen S (eds): "Molecular Basis of Lymphokine Action," Clifton Humana Press, pp 295-311.

Ralph P, Lee MT, Nakoinz I (1989) M-CSF: molecular cloning, structure, *in vitro* and *in vivo* functions. In Sorg C (eds): "Cytokines," Karger S, Basel AG, pp 1-18.

Rambaldi A, Wakamiya N, Vellenga E (1988) Expression of the macrophage colony-stimulating factor and c-fms genes in human actue myeloblastic leukemia cells. J Clin Invest 81:1030-1035.

Rettenmier CW, Roussel MF, Ashmun RA (1987) Synthesis of membrane bound CSF-1 in NIH 3T3 cells transformed by cotransfection of the human CSF-1 and c-fms (CSF-1 receptor) genes. Mol Cell Biol 7:2378-2387.

Ringler GE, Coutifaris C, Strauss III JF, Geier M (1988) Accumulation of colony stimulating factor-1 in amniotic fluid during human pregnancy. Biol Reprod 38(S1):136.

Roberts WM, Look AT, Roussel MF, Sherr CJ (1988) Tandem linkage of human CSF-1 receptor (c-fms) and PDGF receptor genes. Cell 55:655-661.

Roussel MF, Dull TJ, Rettenmier CW (1986) Transforming potential of the c-fms proto-oncogene (CSF-1 receptor). Nature 325:549-551.

Sakai N, Umeda T, Suzuki H, Ishimatsu Y, Shikita M (1987) Macrophage colony-stimulating factor purified from normal human urine. FEBS Lett 222:341-344.

Sampson-Johannes A, Carlino JA (1988) Enhancement of human monocyte tumoricidal activity by recombinant M-CSF. J Immunol 141:3680-3686.

Sechler JMG, Warren MK, Gallin JI (1989) Human non-transformed monocyte-derived macrophage cell lines. J Immunological Meth 119:277-285.

Shadle PJ, Allen JI, Geier MD, Koths K (1989a) Detection of endogenous macrophage colony-stimulating factor (M-CSF) in human blood. Exp Hematol 17:154-159.

Shadle PJ, Aldwin L, Nitecki DE, Koths K (1989b) Human macrophage colony-stimulating factor heterogeneity results from alternative mRNA splicing, differential glycosylation, and proteolytic processing. J Cell Biochem 40:91-107.

Sherr CJ, Rettenmier CW, Sacca R, Roussel MF, Look AT, Stanley ER (1985) The *c-fms* proto-oncogene product is related to the receptor for the mononuclear phagocyte growth factor, CSF-1. Cell 41:665-676.

Stanley ER (1985) The macrophage colony stimulating factor, CSF-1. Meth Enzymol 116:564-587.

Stanley ER, Guilbert LJ, Tushinski RJ (1983) CSF-1, a mononuclear phagocyte lineage-specific hemopoietic growth factor. J Cell Biochem 21:151-159.

Sutherland GR, Baker E, Callen DF (1988) Interleukin-5 is at 5q31 and is deleted in the 5q-syndrome. Blood 71:1150-1152.

Takahashi M, Yeong-Man H, Setsuko Y (1988) Macrophage colony-stimulating factor is produced by human T lymphoblastoid cell line, cem-on: identification by amino-terminal amino acid sequence analysis. Biochem Biophys Res Commun 152:1401-1409.

Tao X, Gao G, Zhang HZ, Zhu DX, Boersma A (1987) Isolation and characterization of human urinary colony-stimulating factor. Biol Chem Hoppe-Seyler 368:187-194.

Troutt AB, Lee F (1989) Tissue distribution of murine hemopoietic growth factor mRNA production. J Cellular Physiology 138:38-44.

Tushinski RJ, Oliver IT, Guilbert LJ (1982) Survival of mononuclear phagocytes depends on a lineage-specific growth factor that the differentiation cells selectively destroy. Cell 28:71-81.

Van de Wijngaert FP, Tas MC, Van der Meer JWM (1987) Growth of osteoclast precursor-like cells from whole mouse bone marrow: inhibitory effect of CSF-1. Bone Miner 3:97-110.

Vellenga E, Rambaldi A, Ernst, TJ, Ostapovicz, Griffin JD (1988) Independent regulation of M-CSF and G-CSF gene expression in human monocytes. Blood 71:1529-1532.

Wang FF, Goldwasser E (1983) Purification of a human urinary colony-stimulating factor. J Cellular Biochem 21:263-275.

Wang LM, Killary AM, Fang XE, Parriott SK, Lalley PA, Bell GI, Sakaguchi AY (1988) Chromosome assignment of mouse insulin, colony stimulating factor 1, and low-density lipoprotein receptors. Genomics 3:172-175.

Warren MK, Ralph P (1986) CSF-1 stimulates human monocyte production of interferon, tumor necrosis factor, and myeloid CSF. J Immunol 137:2281-2285.

Wong GG, Temple PA, Leary AC (1987) Human CSF-1: molecular cloning and expression of 4 kb cDNA encoding the human urinary protein. Science 235:1504-1508.

Young J, Aukerman L, Nachtman J (1989) Pharmacokinetics, efficacy and toxicity of recombinant human M-CSF in rodents and primates. Presented at Clinical Applications of Cytokines, Hannover, Germany.

Hematopoietic Growth Factors
in Transfusion Medicine, pages 65–73

INTERLEUKIN-7: A NEW HEMATOPOIETIC GROWTH FACTOR

Anthony E. Namen, Douglas E. Williams, and
Raymond G. Goodwin

Immunex Corporation

51 University Street, Seattle, WA 98101

INTRODUCTION

The mammalian hematopoietic system is a dynamic and tightly regulated system. Primitive progenitor cells undergo a series of proliferative and differentiative events which ultimately leads to the production of functionally mature effector cells. A large body of *in vitro,* and more recently, *in vivo* evidence suggests that peptide growth factors influence the efflux of cells from the progenitor cell pool to end-stage cells (Broxmeyer and Williams, 1988).

GM-CSF, IL-3, G-CSF, CSF-1 and IL-6 have been shown to be directly stimulatory to myeloid progenitor cells (Broxmeyer and Williams, 1988). Other factors such as IL-1 and IL-4 lack a direct proliferative effect on these progenitors but can enhance the responsiveness to those factors that do promote proliferation. In contrast, the factors which regulate lymphopoiesis at the progenitor cell level are largely unknown despite a large body of evidence showing significant effects of various interleukins on mature T and B cells.

The development of the long-term B lymphoid culture technique by Whitlock and Witte (W/W) (Whitlock and Witte, 1982; Whitlock et al., 1984) was the first demonstration of sustained lymphopoiesis *in vitro.* These cultures gave rise to populations of pro- and pre-B cells over a period of several months. Active cell production was absolutely dependent upon the establishment of a complex stromal cell network which provided the necessary microenvironmental signals or soluble growth factors to promote B-cell genesis. This was demonstrated by the derivation of cell lines from WW cultures which could support pre-B cell growth and produce soluble factors which acted on WW culture derived B cell progenitors (Whitlock, et al., 1987; Hunt, et al., 1987; Namen et al., 1988a). Using the WW culture system, a stromal cell line was developed from which the complementary DNA encoding a pre-B cell stimulatory activity, interleukin-7, (IL-7) was isolated (Namen et al., 1988a).

ISOLATION OF THE IL-7 cDNA

A bioassay to detect soluble factors active on B cell precursors was developed with non-adherent cells derived from WW cultures (Namen et al., 1988a). The target cells in these assays were non-adherent cells isolated from active WW cultures depleted of adherent accessory cells by passage over a Sephadex G-10 column. This population was composed almost entirely of pro- and pre-B cells.

It was well established that stromal cell lines isolated from WW cultures could support the survival and growth of B cell precursors and suggested that such cell lines were a source of potential soluble factors (Whitlock, et al., 1987; Hunt, et al., 1987; Namen et al., 1988a). A stromal cell line was derived in our lab from WW cultures by transfection with a plasmid (PSV3neo) containing the transforming sequences of SV40 using the calcium phosphate procedure (Namen et al., 1988a). The resultant cell lines were screened for production of soluble factors in a thymidine incorporation assay using the aforementioned population of WW cultured B cell precursors, and one clone was identified (IxN/A6) which produced a low level of B cell precursor stimulatory activity.

The IxN/A6 cell line was used as a source of conditioned medium for the biochemical purification of this B cell precursor activity and as a source of mRNA for cDNA library construction and subsequent direct expression cloning (Namen et al., 1988b). A total of 800 L of conditioned medium was purified by a five step procedure of DEAE-Sephacel, SP-Trisacryl, Blue B agarose, reversed phase HPLC, and SDS-PAGE analysis to yield a single protein with a M_r of approximately 25 x 10^3 upon silver staining (Namen et al., 1988a). Simultaneous direct expression cloning studies isolated a single cDNA encoding the B cell precursor activity after screening approximately 720,000 recombinants. Comparison of the predicted amino acid sequence of the protein encoded by this cDNA and the N-terminal amino acid sequence from the biochemically purified protein showed that they were the same molecule (Namen et al., 1988b). This protein was given the designation interleukin-7 (IL-7).

MOLECULAR CHARACTERIZATION OF IL-7

The nucleotide sequence of the cDNA clone containing the murine IL-7 coding sequences was 1,607 base pairs (bp) in length and contained an open reading frame of 462 bp (Namen et al., 1988b). A 548 bp 5' non-coding region preceded the coding sequences and contained eight pseudo-initiation sites upstream from the authentic initiation codon. Removal of this 5' non-coding region from the clone dramatically increased the expression of IL-7 in COS-7 cells and suggested that this region may be involved in regulating expression of IL-7. Murine IL-7 contains a 25 amino acid leader sequence followed by 129 amino acids, giving a predicted molecular mass of ≈14,900. Two potential N-linked glycosylation sites were identified at amino acids 69 and 90 and probably accounts for the difference in the observed M_r of the native molecule and the predicted M_r of 14,900. At least some of the six cysteine residues are involved in intramolecular disulfide bonds as reduction with 2-mercaptoethanol completely inactivates biological activity of the molecule.

The cDNA encoding biologically active human IL-7 was identified by hybridization with the homologous murine clone (Goodwin et al., 1989). A high degree of homology between the murine and human nucleotide sequence exists in the coding region (81%), as well as the 3' (63%) and 5' (73%) non-coding regions. The human cDNA, like the murine cDNA, also possesses eight potential initiation sites in the 5' untranslated region which may be of significance for the regulation of expression of this cytokine. The coding region of the human cDNA is 534 nucleotides in length, coding for a protein of 177 amino acids with a calculated molecular mass of 17,400. Three potential N-linked glycosylation sites are present in the human sequence and the six cysteine residues present in murine IL-7 are present in the human molecule as well. At the amino acid level, a high level of homology (60%) exists between murine and human IL-7 however the predicted sequence of human IL-7 contains a 19 amino acid insert from residues 96-114 not present in the murine homologue. This is due to an additional exon in the human IL-7 gene.

Isolation of polyadenylated mRNA from a variety of human and murine tissues was performed for Northern blot analysis. IL-7 mRNA was detectable in murine spleen, thymus, and liver, and in human spleen and thymus (Namen et al., 1988b; Goodwin et al., 1989). Multiple mRNA species were detected in all tissues and the patterns of RNA species was specific for a given tissue. This heterogeneity in mRNA size may be related to alternative splicing and/or polyadenylation sites.

In Vitro IL-7 BIOLOGY

IL-7 was initially identified as a factor which promoted proliferation, but not differentiation of B cell precursors (Namen et al., 1988a). Both pre- and pro-B cells from WW cultures have been shown to proliferate in response to stimulation by IL-7 (Figure 1). Recently, a clonal assay for pre-B cells in semi-solid cultures has been developed and characterization of the colony forming cell indicated that they were B220$^+$, sIgM$^-$ pre-B cells (Lee et al., 1989). No convincing evidence for differentiation of these cells to sIg$^+$ B cells could be seen within the colonies however an occasional sIg$^+$ cell was seen in <10% of the colonies examined. IL-7 may therefore have weak differentiation promoting ability or, alternatively, the pre-B cells may be programmed to differentiate after a finite number of divisions. Culture of mature B cells from spleen or lymph node demonstrated that IL-7 did not stimulate proliferation of mature B lineage cells.

The high level of IL-7 mRNA in the thymus led to studies of the potential role of IL-7 in T cell development. Unfractionated thymocytes were shown to proliferate in response to IL-7 with a similar half-maximal stimulation level when compared to WW culture derived B cell precursors. Fractionation experiments showed that the most immature T cell precursors, the so called double negatives (CD4$^-$/CD8$^-$), proliferated in response to IL-7 and that this proliferation was a direct response to IL-7 (Conlon et al., 1989a; Watson et al., 1989). The observed proliferation

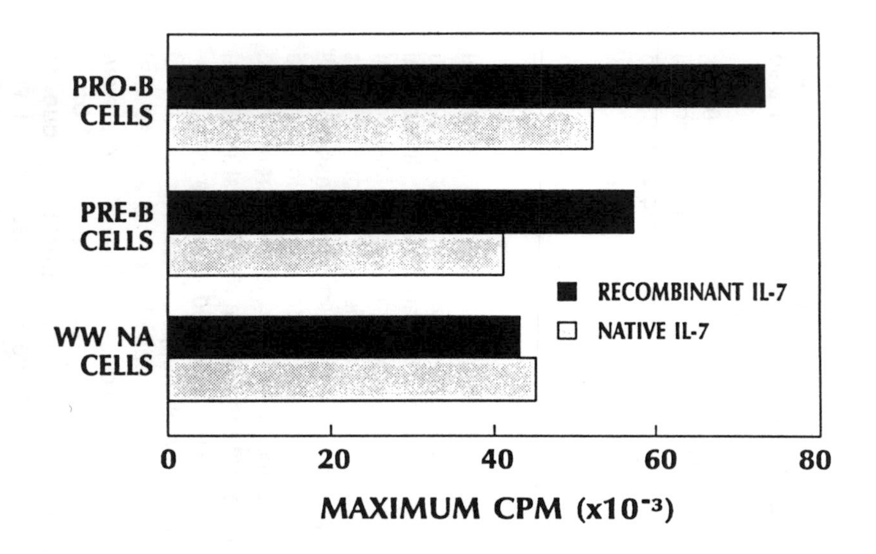

Figure 1: Proliferation of Whitlock Witte (W/W) culture derived B cell precursors in response to saturating concentrations of purified recombinant or native IL-7. Maximum ^{3}H-thymidine incorporation of WW non-adherent cells, $B220^{+}$ pre-B cells, or $B220^{-}$ pro-B cells.

did not result from the secondary production of other known proliferative stimulators such as IL-1, IL-2 or IL-6 (Conlon et al., 1989a). $CD4^-/CD8^-$ cells from either adult thymus or day 13 fetal thymus responded to IL-7 and augmented the response to sub-optimal mitogen levels. Mature peripheral T cells of either the $CD4^+$ or $CD8^+$ phenotype have also been shown to proliferate in response to IL-7, however, only in the presence of sub-optimal mitogen concentrations (Morrissey et al., 1989). With mature T cells, proliferation occurs via induction of IL-2 receptor and subsequent IL-2 production in response to IL-7 plus mitogen and is independent of IL-6. Recent studies indicate that IL-7 can also act synergistically with IL-2 to induce proliferation of $CD4^-/CD8^-$ and $CD4^+/CD8^+$ thymocytes (Conlon et al., 1989b; Williams et al., 1989). This indicates that IL-7 can influence all of the major T cell subpopulations from $CD4^-/CD8^-$ to $CD4^+/CD8^+$ to $CD4^+$ or $CD8^+$ phenotypes (Figure 2).

IN VIVO BIOLOGY OF IL-7

Preliminary pre-clinical studies of IL-7 effects on normal and myelosuppressed mice have shown a dramatic effect on lymphoid and myeloid compartments of treated mice. In normal animals, IL-7 was administered as a twice daily i.p. injection of 500 ng for five days. Animals were sacrificed 1, 3 and 6 days after the cessation of therapy and *in vitro* clonogenic assays, cell surface phenotyping and cellularity determinations were performed. Cellularity was increased in the peripheral blood largely due to the presence of $B220^+$ cells on day 3 post treatment and circulating platelet levels were elevated approximately two-fold on the day after treatment was stopped, returning to normal thereafter. Splenic cellularity was increased two-fold as was that of the mesenteric lymph node. Splenic levels of $sIgM^+$ cells were elevated two-fold and increases were seen in the level of pre-B colony forming cells and CFU-GM, the latter likely due to migration from the bone marrow. Mice were also treated with twice daily IL-7 injections (500 ng/injection) beginning on the day of administration of 750 rads of total body irradiation. IL-7 treatment hastened the recovery of the lymphoid compartments in these mice and reduced the period of thrombocytopenia, suggesting a role in platelet production (Figure 2).

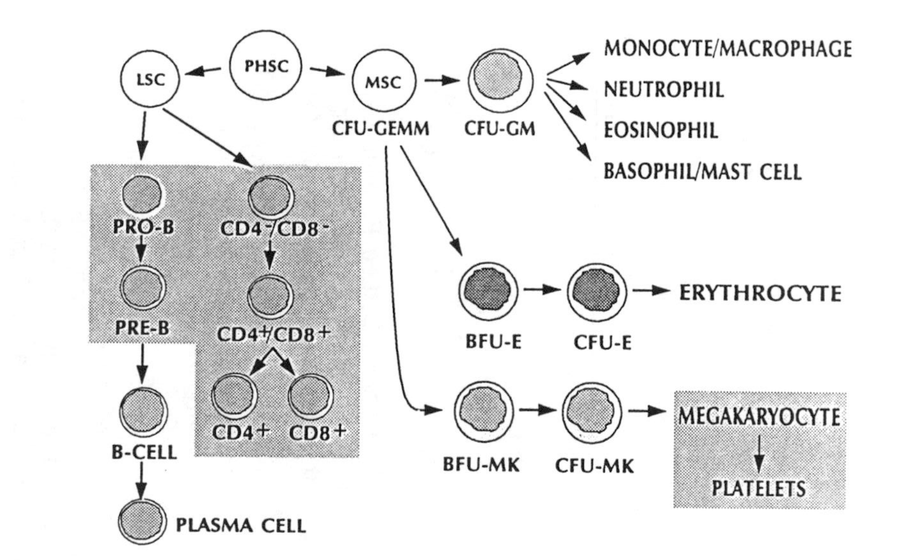

Figure 2: A schematic representation of the hematopoietic hierarchy showing the cells which have been shown to be responsive to IL-7 (stippled area).

PHSC; pluripotential hematopoietic stem cell, LSC; lymphoid stem cell, MSC; myeloid stem cell, CFU-GEMM; mixed myeloid colony forming cell, CFU-GM; granulocyte macrophage progenitor cell, BFU-E; erythroid burst forming cell, CFU-E; erythroid colony forming cell, BFU-MK; megakaryocyte burst forming cell, CFU-MK; megakaryocyte colony forming cell.

SUMMARY

IL-7 is a regulator of early lymphoid progenitors of both the T cell and B cell lineages. The high level of expression of IL-7 mRNA under steady state conditions in the thymus suggest that IL-7 is an important regulator of basal lymphoid development. Early pre-clinical data also suggests that IL-7 may have a role in platelet production.

REFERENCES

Broxmeyer HE, Williams DE (1988). Production of myeloid blood cells and their regulation in health and disease. CRC Crit. Rev. Hematol. Oncol. 8:173.

Conlon PJ, Morrissey PJ, Nordan RP, Grabstein KH, Prickett KS, Reed SG, Goodwin RG, Cosman D, Namen AE (1989a). Murine thymocytes respond to IL-7. Blood, in press.

Conlon PJ, Williams DE, Goodwin RG, Grabstein KH, Widmer MB, Namen AE (1989b). IL-7 synergy with IL-2 in thymic CTL generation. J. Immunol., submitted.

Goodwin RG, Lupton S, Schmierer A, Hjerrild K, Jerzy R, Clevenger W, Gillis S, Cosman D, Namen AE (1989). Human interleukin 7: molecular cloning and growth factor activity on human and murine B-lineage cells. Proc. Natl. Acad. Sci. USA 86:302.

Hunt PA, Robertson D, Weiss D, Rennick D, Lee F, Witte ON (1987). A single bone marrow derived stromal cell type supports the *in vitro* growth of early lymphoid and myeloid cells. Cell 48:997.

Lee G, Namen AE, Gillis S, Ellingsworth L, Kincade PW (1989). Normal B cell precursors responsive to recombinant murine IL-7 and inhibition of IL-7 activity by transforming growth factor-β. J. Immunol. 142:3875.

Morrissey PJ, Goodwin RG, Nordan RP, Anderson D, Grabstein KH, Cosman D, Sims J, Lupton S, Acres B, Reed SG, Mochizuki DY, Eisenman J, Conlon PJ, Namen AE (1989). Recombinant interleukin 7, pre-B cell growth factor, has costimulatory activity on purified mature T cells. J. Exp. Med. 169:707.

Namen AE, Schmierer AE, March CJ, Overell RW, Park LS, Urdal DL, Mochizuki DY (1988). B cell precursor growth-promoting activity. Purification and characterization of a growth factor active on lymphoid progenitors. J. Exp. Med. 167:1988a.

Namen AE, Lupton S, Hjerrild K, Wignall J, Mochizuki DY, Schmierer, A., Mosley, B., March, C. J., Urdal, D., Gillis, S., Cosman, D., and Goodwin, R. G. (1988b). Stimulation of B cell progenitors by cloned murine interleukin-7. Nature 333:6173.

Watson JD, Morrissey PJ, Namen AE, Conlon PJ, Widmer MB (1989). Effect of interleukin-7 on the growth of fetal thymocytes in culture. J. Immunol., in press.

Whitlock CA, Witte ON (1982). Long term culture of B lymphocytes and their precursors from murine bone marrow. Proc. Natl. Acad. Sci. USA 79:3608.

Whitlock CA, Robertson D, Witte ON (1984). Murine B lymphopoiesis in long term culture. J. Immunol. Meth. 6:353.

Whitlock CA, Tidmarsh GF, Muller-Sieburg C, Weissman IL (1987). Bone marrow stromal cell lines with lymphopoietic activity express high levels of a pre-B neoplasia-associated molecule. Cell 48:1009.

Williams DE, Conlon PJ, Smith C, Namen AE, Goodwin RG, Morrissey PJ (1989). Clonal growth of murine thymocytes in semi-solid culture: characterization of the thymocyte colony forming cell (Thy-CFC). J. Exp. Med., submitted.

Hematopoietic Growth Factors
in Transfusion Medicine, pages 75–103

CYTOKINE CONTROL OF HUMAN MEGAKARYOCYTOPOIESIS

Ronald Hoffman, Robert A. Briddell, John E. Straneva, John E. Brandt, Edward Bruno, Arnold Ganser, Norman Hudson, Timothy Guscar

From the Hematology/Oncology Section, Department of Medicine, Indiana University School of Medicine, Indianapolis, IN 46202 and the Department of Hematology, University of Frankfurt, FRG.

INTRODUCTION

During the past decade, advances in protein purification and gene cloning have been applied to the isolation and characterization of hematopoietic growth factors (Clark et al., 1987; Metcalf et al., 1985). The adoption of such methodologies has led to many new insights into the means by which cytokines control blood cell production (Clark et al., 1987; Metcalf et al., 1985). Recently these new tools have been applied to the study of megakaryocytopoiesis, resulting in important advances. The information obtained from these studies will be reviewed here.

Humoral Regulation of Megakaryocytopoiesis

Studies in a variety of animal models suggest that platelet production can be altered by humoral factors (Odell et al., 1961; Ebbe et al., 1968; Adams et al., 1978; Levin et al., 1979; Ebbe et al., 1988; Harker et al., 1968; Young et al., 1987). Induction of thrombocytopenia in the rodent either by the use of an antiplatelet antiserum or exchange transfusion with platelet poor blood is accompanied by increases in marrow megakaryocyte numbers, size, and DNA content; thrombocytosis created by platelet transfusions results in reciprocal changes in the same megakaryocyte parameters (Odell et al., 1961; Young et al., 1987;

McDonald et al., 1988). A large number of such studies performed by a number of investigators have provided an impetus to characterize and purify the cytokines responsible for in vivo platelet production (Odell et al., 1961; Ebbe et al., 1968; Adams et al., 1978; Levin et al., 1979, Ebbe et al., 1988; Harker et al., 1968; Young et al., 1987). Many laboratories have sought to characterize a so called thrombocytopoiesis stimulating factor (TSF or thrombopoietin), which would be a candidate molecule for being the primary regulator of platelet production. Workers have referred to such a molecule as megakaryocyte potentiator activity, thrombocytopoiesis stimulating factor, thrombopoietin, or megakaryocyte stimulating factor (McDonald et al., 1985; Hill et al., 1987; Evatt et al., 1974, Sparrow et al., 1987, Swee-Huat 1986). Although it is still uncertain whether such a pivotal molecule exists, lessons learned from the studies of other hematopoietic lineages would suggest that even if such a thrombopoietin is a reality, a variety of other cytokines would also be expected to be capable of altering platelet production (Sieff et al., 1987).

Intuitively, one would expect that a process so vital to survival as platelet production would be regulated by cytokines exclusively responsible for this process. The hypothesis that megakaryocyte/platelet specific growth factors exist has provided the basis for over twenty-five years of work and although this hypothesis is likely correct, it is to date unproven. With the availability of a growing number of recombinant cytokines originally thought to affect predominantly single hematopoietic lineages, but now known to affect multiple hematopoietic lineages including megakaryocytopoiesis, the confirmation of the existence of megakaryocyte specific growth factors remains an important effort (Sieff et al., 1987). This question will only be adequately answered when the responsible cytokines are purified, their amino acid sequences determined, and their uniqueness established. Until these goals are accomplished, reports of megakaryocyte specific cytokines should be interpreted with cautious optimism.

Regulation of a number of cellular systems has been shown to be due not only to simulators of cellular proliferation but also to inhibitors. The possibility that such negative regulators of megakaryocytopoiesis might be operational during megakaryocytopoiesis was initially raised by the studies of Vainchenker et al., Messner et al., Kimura et al., and Solberg et al., (Messner et al., 1982; Solberg et al., 1985; Kimura et al., 1984; Vainchenker et al., 1982). These workers independently observed that _in vitro_ megakaryocyte colony formation was improved when human plasma, rather than serum, was used as a culture constituent in megakaryocyte progenitor cell (CFU-MK) assays. The suggestion by these investigators that platelets might be the source of inhibitors of CFU-MK proliferation has provided the basis for attempts to identify such inhibitor molecules (Messner et al., 1982; Solberg et al., 1985; Kimura et al., 1984; Vainchenker et al., 1982).

Megakaryocyte Colony Stimulating Factor

Urine, serum, and plasma obtained from patients with hypomegakaryocytic thrombocytopenia have been shown to be capable of promoting the formation of megakaryocytic colonies _in vitro_ (Hoffman et al., 1981; Kawakita et al., 1981; Kawakita et al., 1983; Mazur et al., 1985; Mazur et al., 1984; Geibler et al., 1985). Whether this MK-CSA is due to the presence of a single unique megakaryocyte colony stimulating factor (MK-CSF) or a combination of several cytokines with MK-CSA is presently unknown. Data have been provided by several laboratories suggesting that the elaboration of MK-CSA in human plasma or serum is not directly related to platelet numbers but rather inversely related to megakaryocyte mass (Hoffman et al., 1981; Kawakita et al., 1983; Williams et al., 1982; Mazur et al., 1981). The elaboration of MK-CSA has been observed in a variety of clinical disorders including selective amegakaryocytic thrombocytopenia, aplastic anemia, and marrow hypocellularity following cytotoxic chemotherapy or chemoradiotherapy in preparation for allogeneic marrow transplantation (Hoffman et al., 1981; Kawakita et al., 1981; Kawakita et al., 1983; Mazur et al., 1985; Mazur et al., 1984; Geibler et al., 1985; Yamasaki et al., 1988; de Alarcon et al., 1988). Miura et al., have developed a small animal model which provides an opportunity to define the relationship between platelet numbers and detectability of MK-CSA (Miura et al., 1988). These investigators compared assayable MK-CSA in plasma of severely thrombocytopenic rats following irradiation to that detected in similarly irradiated animals who received platelet transfusions in order to maintain normal platelet numbers (Miura et al., 1988). Assayable MK-CSA was equally elevated in each of these experimental groups as compared to animals which were not irradiated (Miura et al., 1988). This work is in agreement with the hypothesis that MK-CSA elaboration occurs independently of platelet numbers.

The cytokines responsible for plasma MK-CSA in hypomegakaryocytic individuals must be identified in order to understand the contribution of various growth factors to CFU-MK regulation in vivo. The biochemical purification of each of these cytokines has recently been pursued by a number of laboratories and has resulted in limited success. A number of sources of MK-CSA, including aplastic anemia urine, selective amegakaryocytic thrombocytopenia plasma, or thrombocytopenic plasma, obtained following the administration of sublethal irradiation to dogs, have each been used as starting materials for these purification procedures (Kawakita et al., 1983; Hoffman et al., 1985; Abe et al., 1988). An immortalized cell line, which elaborates MK-CSA and which would potentially serve as a ready source of this cytokine, has not been identified. The purification of a number of other cytokines has clearly been expedited by the availability of cell lines elaborating the biological activities of interest (Clark et al., 1987; Metcalf et al., 1985). The lack of access to such a cell line has surely hindered MK-CSF purification efforts.

Characterization of partially purified preparations of MK-CSF have resulted in the assignment of a variety of molecular weights to this cytokine (Kawakita et al., 1983; Hoffman et al., 1985; Abe et al., 1988). In our laboratory, a polyclonal rabbit antiserum which neutralizes MK-CSA present in human plasma was developed (Yang et al., 1986). This antiserum did not neutralize the MK-CSA of IL-3 or GM-CSF but did neutralize MK-CSA in a protein fraction partially purified from human plasma (Yang et al., 1986; Straneva et al., 1987; Straneva et al., 1988). In addition, Mazur et al. recently reported that IL-3 and GM-CSF neutralizing antibodies did not diminish the MK-CSA present in plasma obtained from thrombocytopenic dogs or humans (Mazur et al., 1988). These data collectively indicate the presence of an additional cytokine(s) besides GM-CSF or IL-3 in human plasma exhibiting MK-CSA. Although data from our laboratory had initially indicated that the MK-CSF was purified to homogeneity, further studies of this preparation have conclusively shown that this material was not at a level of purity to allow for accurate amino acid sequencing. It is hoped that further information about these molecules will be generated in our own laboratory and that of others in the near future.

Other Cytokines Affecting CFU-MK Proliferation

Determination of the range of activities of the purified and recombinant cytokines already isolated have indicated that these cytokines can affect in vitro and in vivo megakaryocytopoiesis (Quesenberry et al., 1985; Robinson et al., 1987; Mazur et al., 1987; Kaushansky et al., 1986; Sieff et al., 1987; Lopez et al., 1987; Peschel et al., 1987; Dukes et al., 1986; Clark et al., 1986; Mizoguchi et al., 1986; Williams et al., 1984; Bruno et al., 1989; Muzure et al., 1988; Bruno et al., 1988; Teramura et al., 1988; McNiece et al., 1988; Wong et al., 1988; Messner et al., 1987; Donahue et al., 1988; Donahue et al., 1986; Krumwieh et al., 1988; Krumwieh et al., 1989; Ganser et al., 1989; Wong et al., 1988; Ikebuchi et al., 1987; McGrath et al., 1989; Bruno et al., 1989; Ishibashi et al., 1989). Some of these cytokines actually have MK-CSA while others act in synergy with other factors to affect CFU-MK proliferation.

Data generated in a large number of laboratories are in agreement that recombinant GM-CSF and IL-3 both individually have MK-CSA in addition to their ability to affect a number of other hematopoietic lineages (Quesenberry et al., 1985; Robinson et al., 1987; Mazur et al., 1987; Kaushansky et al., 1986; Sieff et al., 1987; Lopez et al., 1987; Teramura et al., 1988; McNiece et al., 1988; Wong et al., 1988; Messner et al., 1987; Donahue et al., 1988; Donahue et al., 1986; Krumwieh et al., 1988; Krumwieh et al., 1989). With regard to their MK-CSA, IL-3 appears to have the ability to promote the formation of greater numbers of megakaryocyte colonies than GM-CSF (Quesenberry et al., 1985; Messner et al., 1987). In addition, the effects of GM-CSF and IL-3 are additive in that colony formation by a combination of the two growth factors approximates the sum of colony formation by each growth factor alone (Robinson et al., 1987; Bruno et al., 1988; Krumwieh et al., 1988). These cytokines not only increase colony formation, but also increase the number of cells comprising individual CFU-MK derived colonies (Bruno et al., 1988). Recently, continuous infusions of human IL-3 in a primate model has reported to result in profound increases in mean platelet counts (Krumwieh et al., 1988; Krumwieh et al., 1989). Administration of rGM-CSF to primates also has resulted in modest, albeit, inconsistent effects on platelet numbers (Donahue et al., 1986). Krumwieh et al. have further explored the in vivo action of these cytokines by administering them in sequence (Krumwieh et al., 1988; Krumwieh et al., 1989). Primates were first injected with interleukin-3 and then subsequently with GM-CSF (Krumwieh et al., 1988; Eschbach et al., 1987). Such priming with IL-3 followed by GM-CSF administration resulted in a dose-dependent significant increase in platelet numbers even though IL-3 and GM-CSF alone, at the doses administered, had no significant influence on platelet numbers (Krumwieh et al., 1988). These data suggest that GM-CSF and IL-3 not only have an additive effective on megakaryocytopoiesis in vitro but also in vivo. Data has recently been presented which indicates that rIL-3 administered to patients with a variety of disorders of thrombopoiesis leads to remarkable increases in circulating platelet numbers (Ganser et al., 1989). These preliminary studies indicate that rIL-3 may be a promising pharmacological agent for the treatment of thrombocytopenic disorders.

Another recombinant cytokine, IL-6, has recently been shown to also possess MK-CSA. IL-6, a human B cell stimulating factor, was originally characterized as a T cell derived factor that promoted the terminal maturation of activated B cells to immunoglobulin-producing cells (Wong et al., 1988). This cytokine has been shown to be identical to B_2 interferon, 26kd protein, and hybridoma growth factor (Wong et al., 1988). Recently, Wong et al. and Ikebuchi et al. have shown that rIL-6 has MK-CSA; this work has been confirmed in our own laboratory and that of McGrath et al. (Wong et al., 1988; Ikebuchi et al., 1987; McGrath et al., 1989; Bruno et al., 1989). IL-6 appears, however, to be less effective than either rIL-3 or rGM-CSF in promoting megakaryocyte colony formation (Bruno et al., 1989). In addition, Ishibashi et al. have presented data to indicate that rIL-6 is a potent stimulator of MK maturation (Ishibashi et al., 1989). Such data has led to speculations that IL-6 might be closely related to thrombopoietin.

Examination of the effect of erythropoietin on megakaryocytopoiesis has been prompted by the clinical observations that anemic states are frequently accompanied by thrombocytosis. McDonald et al. recently reported that administering 2.0 - 7.5 units of recombinant erythropoietin/mouse did not stimulate platelet production, but that larger doses (15 units/mouse administered over 2 days) lead to a significant stimulation of thrombopoiesis as determined by radioactive selenomethionine incorporation into platelets (McDonald et al., 1987). Platelet counts were still not, however, elevated in these animals (McDonald et al., 1987). Berridge et al. have reported an actual increase in platelet numbers following erythropoietin administration to rodents (Berrisge et al., 1988). The clinical relevance of such reports are questionable since in several clinical trials in which the effects of recombinant erythropoietin therapy in patients with chronic renal failure were tested, no significant elevation of platelets at the doses of erythropoietin administered was observed (Winerls et al., 1986; Eschbach et al., 1987).

The effect of erythropoietin on CFU-MK proliferation has also been extensively analyzed with conflicting results. Using partially purified erythropoietin preparations, a number of laboratories have reported that erythropoietin has MK-CSA, while an equal number have failed to confirm this effect (Clark et al., 1986; Vainchenker et al., 1974; Mazur et al., 1981; Sakaguchi et al., 1987; Dessypris et al., 1987; Lu et al., 1988; Williams et al., 1979; Rossi et al., 1989). One explanation for this inconsistency of results might be due to contamination of the partially purified erythropoietin preparations with other cytokines. Both Vainchenker et al. and Williams et al. however, using highly purified preparations of erythropoietin (70,000 units/mg protein), were able to detect erythropoietin's MK-CSA (Williams et al., 1984; Vainchenker et al., 1974). In addition, Sakaguchi et al. using a serum-free assay system reported that high concentrations of recombinant erythropoietin (10 units/ml) were capable of promoting megakaryocyte colony formation (Sakaguchi et al., 1987). Dessypris et al. however, found that although recombinant erythropoietin itself had no MK-CSA, it did increase megakaryocyte colony formation in the presence of phytohemagglutinin stimulated leukocyte conditioned media (PHA-LCM) or serum (Dessypris et al., 1987). This group has presented data that factors present in PHA-LCM and human serum are absolutely required for recombinant erythropoietin to exert its effect on the CFU-MK. The hypothesis that recombinant erythropoietin might require the presence of other cytokines to have MK-CSA has been confirmed by the work of Peschel et al. and Bruno et al. (Peschel et al., 1987; Krumwieh et al., 1989). Perhaps the best perspective on the role of erythropoietin in the regulation of erythropoiesis is provided by the report of Rossi et al. (Rossi et al., 1989). Their data suggests that erythropoietin has little influence on megakaryocytopoiesis at the doses known to elicit a maximal erythropoietic response. They suggest that although subsets of murine splenic megakaryocyte progenitors may be influenced by extraordinarily high doses of erythropoietin it is unlikely that this phenomenon is a significant factor in the overall regulation of megakaryocytopoiesis (Rossi et al., 1989). Data obtained in several laboratories suggest that several cytokines, IL-1, thrombopoietin, and G-CSF by themselves do not have MK-CSA (Bruno et al., 1989; Bruno et al., 1988). These cytokines have been shown only to affect CFU-MK cloning efficiency when assayed in combination with other growth factors. Thrombopoietin, for instance, has a synergistic relationship with IL-1 alpha (Krumwieh et al., 1988). While IL-1 alpha and thrombopoietin individually have no MK-CSA, various combinations of these growth factors are able to promote megakaryocyte colony formation (Krumwieh et al., 1989). Williams et al. demonstrated that while partially purified thrombopoietin did not directly stimulate megakaryocyte colony formation, it acted together with WEHI-3 conditioned media, a source of IL-3, to augment _in vitro_ megakaryocyte colony formation (Williams et al., 1979). Recently, Bruno et al. have shown that the addition of thrombopoietin to suboptimal concentrations of rIL-3 resulted in an increased cloning efficiency of human CFU-MK (Krumwieh et al., 1989). By contrast, the addition of thrombopoietin to rGM-CSF containing assays actually decreased the MK-CSA of rGM-CSF. Erythropoietin also appears to potentiate the MK-CSA of IL-3 and rGM-CSF by promoting the formation of greater numbers of mixed colonies containing megakaryocytes (Bruno et al., 1989). In addition, McNiece et al. have shown that although rG-CSF has no MK-CSA, it is capable of increasing the number of megakaryocyte colonies formed in the presence of rIL-3 as compared to assays containing rIL-3 alone (McNiece et al., 1988).

These findings indicate that many cytokines may contribute to the regulation of _in vitro_ human megakaryocytopoiesis. Since heterogeneous cell populations were used as a source of target cells in many of these studies, it is possible that some of the observed effects are the consequence of cytokines acting indirectly by stimulating marrow accessory cells to elaborate factors which then directly influence the CFU-MK, rather than all of these cytokines directly affecting the CFU-MK. There is some precedence for this hypothesis. The effect of IL-1 alpha and tumor necrosis factor on hematopoiesis, for instance, have been in part attributed to their ability to cause either stromal cells, fibroblasts, endothelial cells, or T-lymphocytes to elaborate a number of cytokines including GM-CSF, IL-3, G-CSF or IL-6, which might then directly influence hematopoietic progenitor cell proliferation (Zucali et al., 1986; Munker et al., 1986; Koeffler et al., 1987; Sieff et al., 1988; Yang et al., 1988).

Inhibitors of Megakaryocyte Colony Formation

The observation that plasma is superior to serum as a culture constituent in supporting megakaryocyte colony formation has suggested that platelets might elaborate or contain inhibitors of megakaryocyte colony formation (Messmer et al., 1982; Solberg et al., 1985; Kimura et al., 1984; Vainchenker et al., 1982). Several laboratories are now actively working to identify serum constituents that might be responsible for this inhibitory activity (Dessypris et al., 1987; Mitjavila et al., 1988; Gewirtz et al., 1989; Ganser et al., 1987; Breton-Gorius et al., 1987). Solberg et al., Ishibashi et al., and Mitjavila et al. have all reported that transforming growth factor beta (TGF beta), a cytokine found in relatively high concentrations in platelets, might be in part responsible for this inhibitory activity (Solberg et al., 1985; Ishibashi et al., 1987; (Mitjavila et al., 1988). The effects of TGF-beta, however are not limited to the megakaryocyte lineage (Mitjavila et al., 1988). TGF-beta has a similar effect on a number of other hematopoietic and nonhematopoietic cell types (Mitjavila et al., 1985). TGF-beta might not be the only platelet constituent with such inhibitory action. Dessypris et al. have partially purified a platelet released glycoprotein with a molecular weight of 12-17k daltons, which appears to have a different biological range of activities than TGF-beta (Dessypris et al., 1987). This platelet released glycoprotein has been reported to be a specific inhibitor of the CFU-MK and not to affect in vitro granulopoiesis or erythropoiesis (Dessypris et al., 1987). Mitjavila et al. and Gewirtz et al. have also shown that platelet factor-4, a megakaryocyte/platelet alpha granule constituent, inhibits megakaryocyte colony formation but not erythroid or granulocyte/macrophage colony formation (Mitjavila et al., 1988; Gewirtz et al., 1989). However, Dessypris et al. and Gewritz et al. have suggested that the particular inhibitory molecule that they have identified primarily affects megakaryocyte maturation and not CFU-MK proliferation (Mitjavila et al., 1988; Gewirtz et al., 1989). The relationship between the platelet released glycoprotein identified by Dessypris et al, TGF-Beta and PF-4 will require purification of this activity to homogeneity in order to determine if it is indeed a novel cytokine.

Ganser et al. have indicated that cytokines not produced by megakaryocytes and platelets can also inhibit megakaryocyte colony formation. They have reported that recombinant interferon alpha and gamma are both capable of inhibiting megakaryocyte colony formation (Ganser et al., 1987). The mechanisms underlying this inhibition appear to be different since interferon alpha directly affects the CFU-MK while interferon gamma's action is reported to be mediated through an accessory cell population (Ganser et al., 1987).

Regulators of Megakaryocyte Maturation

Maturation of megakaryocytes from immature, largely non-DNA synthesizing cells to morphologically identifiable megakaryocytes involves a number of processes including the appearance of cytoplasmic organelles, the acquisition of membrane antigens and glycoproteins, and the release of platelets (Breton-Gorius et al., 1987). A number of cytokines are now known to act as promoters or inhibitors of this maturation process.

A lineage specific promotor of megakaryocyte maturation, a so-called thrombopoietin, has been detected in thrombocytopenic rodent and human plasma (Odell et al., 1961; McDonald et al., 1985). Purification of this thrombopoietin has been an ongoing project in a large number of laboratories for over three decades (McDonald et al., 1985; Hill et al., 1987; Evatt et al., 1974; Sparrow et al., 1987; Swee-Huat et al., 1986; Sieff et al., 1987; Tayrien et al., 1987). While a broad range of biological activities have been attributed to thrombopoietin, it is not certain to date that these activities are due to only one cytokine. Partially purified preparations of thrombopoietin are capable of accelerating cytoplasmic maturation of megakaryocytes, promoting megakaryocyte protein synthesis and stimulating endomitosis in immature megakaryocytes (Odell et al., 1961; Ebbe et al., 1968; Adams et al., 1978; Levin et al., 1979; Ebbe et al., 1988; Harker et al., 1968; Young et al., 1987; McDonald et al., 1988; McDonald et al., 1985; Hill et al., 1987; Evatt et al., 1974; Sparrow et al., 1987; Swee-Huat et al., 1986; Sieff et al., 1987). Thrombopoietin by itself has little MK-CSA, but is able to influence CFU-MK proliferation by interacting with several cytokines including IL-1 and IL-3 to increase *in vitro* megakaryocyte colony formation (Bruno et al., 1989). Conclusive data that *in vivo* administration of thrombopoietin will result in elevations in platelet numbers are presently not available. Lack of availability of adequate amounts of purified thrombopoietin to perform such critical studies has prevented the performance of these much-needed experiments. A numbers of investigators have attempted to purify thrombopoietin from a variety of sources including rabbit thrombocytopenic plasma, human embryonic kidney cell conditioned media, and urine gathered from severely thrombocytopenic patients (McDonald et al., 1985; Hill et al., 1987; Evatt et al., 1974; Sparrow et al., 1987; Swee-Huat et al., 1986; Tayrien et al., 1987). Thrombopoietin has been reported to be a glycoprotein with an assigned molecular weight of between 15-48,000 daltons (McDonald et al., 1985). Discrepancies in molecular weight with assignments may be due to the propensity of this molecule to aggregate under denaturing conditions (McDonald et al., 1988). Tayrien and Rosenberg have reported that a thrombopoietin-like molecule isolated from both rabbit thrombocytopenic plasma and human embryonic kidney cell conditioned media have similar properties and are likely identical molecules (Tayrien et al., 1987).

A number of groups have performed experiments to show that thrombopoietin is a unique molecule. Using an antiserum which neutralizes human MK-CSF, Straneva and co-workers have demonstrated that the thrombopoietin-like material present in aplastic anemia serum is immunologically distinct from MK-CSF (Straneva et al., 1987). Conversely, an anti-thrombopoietin antiserum did not neutralize the MK-CSA of aplastic anemia serum but did negate its ability to accelerate megakaryocyte maturation (Straneva et al., 1988). In addition, based on the characteristic binding of thrombopoietin and erythropoietin to a variety of lectin affinity columns, erythropoietin and thrombopoietin have been shown to be distinct molecules (Hill et al., 1987; Spivak et al., 1977). Several groups have, however, presented data which suggests that IL-6 and thrombopoietin might be related molecules (Ishibashi et al., 1989). Two laboratories have recently claimed to have purified homogenous preparations of thrombopoietin (McDonald et al., 1985; Tayrien et al., 1987). The uniqueness of these preparations will only be confirmed with amino acid sequencing.

Thrombopoietin physiology is also not well defined. The elaboration of thrombopoietin-like activities has been shown to be inversely related to peripheral platelet numbers (McDonald et al., 1985; McDonald et al., 1988). The site of production of thrombopoietin production or function in the production of disease states in man are as yet not well established (Young et al., 1987; McDonald et al., 1988).

Clinical Disorders of Thrombopoiesis

We have recently reported a patient with acquired cyclic amegakaryocytic thrombocytopenia in whom we were able to implicate an abnormality of cytokine function in the pathobiology of her hematological disorder (Hoffman et al., 1989). The ability of the patient's low density marrow cells to form megakaryocyte colonies in the presence of varying concentrations of rGM-CSF or rIL-3 was tested. In the presence of each of these cytokines, normal numbers of CFU-MK derived colonies were observed, even though there were no megakaryocytes detected when this marrow specimen was examined morphologically. The patient's marrow cells formed normal numbers of colonies derived from other hematopoietic progenitor cells. A complement dependent or independent cytoxic antibody directed against the patient's CFU-MK was next sought as an explanation for the patient's amegakaryocyte

Table 1

Effect of Prior Treatment of Autologous Marrow Cells with Patient's Immunoglobulin Fraction on Megakaryocytic Colony Formation

Prior Treatment	CFU-MK/2 x 10^5 cells plated [1]
Control I	30.5 ± 3.5[2]
Patient Ig	25.0 ± 5.6
Complemen	26.5 ± 4.9
Control Ig + Complement	25.0 ± 7.0
Patient Ig + Complement	23.5 ± 6.3[3]

[1] Each aliquot of cells were exposed to the above listed condition, washed and then plated in the presence of 100 units/ml of recombinant IL-3.

[2] Each point represents the mean ± SD of duplicate assays.

[3] $p > 0.05$

thrombocytopenia. Exposure of autologous marrow cells to the patient's Ig fraction in the presence or absence of complement failed to cause a statistically significant decrease in colony formation.

The hypothesis that the patient's clinical disorder could be due to an inhibitor which altered the ability of a cytokine to promote megakaryocyte colony formation was next tested. The ability of patient serum or control serum to alter cytokine promoted progenitor cell derived colony formation was assessed. Neither the patient's serum nor control serum affected the ability of rIL-3 or rGM-CSF to promote the formation of BFU-E, CFU-GM, or CFU-GEMM derived colonies. By contrast, patient serum markedly diminished the capacity of rGM-CSF, but not rIL-3 to promote megakaryocyte colony formation. The GM-CSF blocking action was localized to an IgG enriched fraction of the patient's serum. By contrast, other Ig fractions from the patient containing IgM or IgA did not contain any GM-CSF blocking activity. In Table 2 the ability of patient IgG to block the capacity of rGM-CSF or rIL-3 to promote megakaryocyte colony formation by autologous, freshly thawed, cryopreserved marrow cells is shown. Again, the patient's IgG blocked the action rGM-CSF but not rIL-3.

Table 2

Effect of Patient IgG Fraction on GM-CSF and IL-3 Promoted Megakaryocyte Colony Formation by Autologous Freshly Thawed Cryopreserved Marrow Cells

Addition to Culture	CFUI/MK2 x 10^5 Cells Plated
None	1.5 ± 0.7[1]
Recombinant GM-CSF (10 units/ml)	26.0 ± 0.0
Recombinant IL-3 (100 units/ml)	26.5 ± 3.5
Recombinant GM-CSF + IgG	3.0 ± 0.0[2]
Recombinant IL-3 + IgG	28.5 ± 4.9

[1] Each point represents the mean ± SD of duplicate assays.

[2] $p < 0.05$

Increasing concentrations of rGM-CSF were added to overcome the GM-CSF blocking action of the patient's serum. Even by increasing the rGM-CSF concentration by 10-fold, the blocking action of the patient's serum could not be overcome. In addition, if normal human marrow cells were exposed to normal IgG or patient IgG fraction for 1 hour, washed and plated in the presence of either GM-CSF or IL-3, the subsequent ability of GM-CSF, but not IL-3, to promote megakaryocyte colony was prevented. When normal LD marrow cells were exposed to rGM-CSF for 1-4 hours under the experimental conditions described and then plated in the presence of rGM-CSF and the patient's IgG fraction, the blocking action of the patient's IgG

Table 3

Effect of Increasing Concentrations of Recombinant GM-CSF on the GM-CSF Blocking Action of the Patients Serum

Addition to Culture[1]	CFU-MK/2 x 10^5 Cells Plated
None	1.5 ± 0.7[2]
10 units/ml rGM-CSF	17.0 ± 2.8
10 units/ml rGM-CSF + Patient Serum	5.0 ± 0.03
25 units/ml rGM-CSF + Patient Serum	5.5 ± 2.1[3]
50 units/ml rGM-CSF + Patient Serum	8.5 ± 0.7[3]
100 units/ml rGM-CSF + Patient Serum	6.0 ± 1.4[3]

[1] Low density normal marrow cells were plated in the presence of varying concentrations of rGM-CSF and a constant percentage of patient serum (5%).

[2] Each point represents the mean ± SD of assays performed in duplicate. Similar results were obtained in one additional study.

[3] $p < 0.02$.

fraction was no longer detectable. Since low density marrow cells constitute a heterogeneous cell population, the possibility existed that the cellular target of the GM-CSF blocking antibody was either the CFU-MK itself or a marrow accessory cell which secondarily releases a cytokine which promotes megakaryocyte colony formation.

To resolve this issue, a population of marrow cells enriched for CFU-MK was used as a cellular target for the rGM-CSF blocking IgG fraction. These data indicate that the ability of rGM-CSF but not rIL-3 to promote megakaryocyte colony formation by $CD34^+DR^+$ marrow could be blocked by the patient's IgG fraction but not control IgG fraction (Table 4).

Cyclical hematopoietic deficiencies are rare events in man. They are characterized by regular predictable oscillations of cellular elements of the blood. Perhaps, the best known of these entities is human cyclic neutropenia, which is associated with fever, malaise, aphthous stomatitis, and mucous membrane infections occurring at the time of neutrophil Nadir (Wright et al., 1981).

Table 4

Effect of the Patient IgG Fraction on Megakaryocyte Colony Formation by Highly Enriched Fractions of Normal Human Marrow Cells

Addition to Culture	CFU-MK/10^4 $CD34^+DR^+$ Cells Plated
None	3.8 ± 1.1[1]
IL-3 (100 units/ml)	16.0 ± 1.4
GM-CSF (10 units/ml)	17.5 ± 2.1
IL-3 + Patient IgG	15.5 ± 2.1
GM-CSF + Patient IgG	8.0 ± 1.4[2]

[1] Each point represents the mean ± SD of duplicate assays performed on two separate occasions.

[2] $p < 0.05$. These findings indicate that the CFU-MK itself is the likely cellular target for the GM-CSF blocking antibody.

Manifestations of this disease usually begin in childhood, although in about 25% of patients the symptoms occur after age 20 (Wright et al., 1981; Loughran et al., 1986). The adult onset of the cyclic amegakaryocytic in our patient is therefore, most reminiscent of adult type cyclic neutropenia. The precise etiology of cyclic neutropenia is unknown, although the defect appears to reside at the progenitor cell level (Wright et al., 1981; Loughran et al., 1986). Studies by Loughran et al. have indicated that the adult onset cyclic neutropenia may be distinguished morphologically from the more common childhood onset cyclic neutropenia by the presence of increased numbers of circulating large granular lymphocytes (Loughran et al., 1986). At no time were large granular lymphocytes observed in our patient's peripheral blood or marrow.

Cyclical hematopoiesis is not limited to abnormalities in the neutrophil lineage. In fact, a strain of grey collie dogs is known to have spontaneous cycles of the number of granulocytes, monocytes, reticulocytes, and platelets (Jones et al., 1975). Cyclical thrombocytopenia is an extremely rare disorder in man characterized by regular fluctuations in platelets (Cohen et al., 1974; Mentiove et al., 1987). Platelet cycles often occur in synchrony with menstruation, but exceptions to this pattern have been described, and the condition has been reported in otherwise normal men (Engstrom et al., 1966; Wasastjema et al., 1967; Menitove et al., 1987). It is generally thought that cyclic thrombocytopenia results from periodic failure of effective platelet production. Some reports have, however, suggested that accelerated platelet destruction may also be an important pathogenetic element (Mentiove et al., 1987; Menitove et al., 1987; Tomer et al., 1988). Platelet reactive autoantibodies have recently been demonstrated in patients with cyclic thrombocytopenia (Mentiove et al., 1987; Menitove et al., 1987). Menitove et al. reported two patients with this disorder with platelet counts varying between 1 and 900 x 10^9 during 10-25 day cycles (Mentiove et al., 1987; Menitove et al., 1987). These investigators found an inverse relationship between the number of platelets and the amount of platelet surface IgG or plasma platelet bindable IgG detected. These findings indicate that cyclical production of an autoantibody might cause the periodic destruction of platelets (Mentiove et al., 1987; Menitove et al., 1987). Reticuloendothelial function may, however, also be an important determinant of platelet destruction. Tomer et al., recently reported studies of two women with cyclic thrombocytopenia (Tomer et al., 1988). These studies indicated that periodic fluctuations in the ability of the reticuloendothelial system to recognize and destroy sensitized platelets led to the cyclical nature of this disorder (Tomer et al., 1988). The lack of detectable platelet associated IgG or serum antiplatelet antibodies in our patient, however, makes it unlikely that her disorder was due to an immune mediated destruction of platelets (Hoffman et al., 1989).

The data presented in this report suggests that the patients IgG fraction might perturb megakaryocytopoiesis by blocking or inactivating the GM-CSF receptor. Autoantibodies to cell surface receptors have been previously implicated as etiological factors in myasthenia gravis (Doniach et al., 1982; Drachman et al., 1982), allergic rhinitis and asthma (Venter et al., 1980; Fraser et al., 1981), insulin resistant diabetes associated with acanthosis nigricans (Kahn et al., 1976), and rare cases of iron deficiency due to anti-transferrin receptor antibodies (Larrick et al., 1981). Studies by Weissman et al. in which the human leukemia cell line K562 was treated with an anti-transferrin receptor monoclonal antibody provide a model which might be utilized to explain the disorder observed in our patient (Weissman et al., 1986). Treatment of the cell line with this monoclonal antibody resulted in reduction of the number of transferrin receptors on K562 cells that participate in iron uptake (Weissman et al., 1986). This reduction in receptor members was in part due to enhanced degradation transferrin receptor (Clark et al., 1987; McDonald et al., 1988). A similar reduction of receptor number has been observed upon treatment of receptor bearing target tissues with other anti-receptor antibodies (Granfeld et al., 1989; Stoscheck et al., 1989). Exposure of the CFU-MK to the GM-CSF blocking IgG fraction might result in a reduction of GM-CSF receptors, leading to decreased sensitivity to GM-CSF and eventually thrombocytopenia. It is also possible that the patient's antibody recognizes a site distinct from the GM-CSF binding site. Autoantibodies to isolated and solubilized acetylcholine receptors (Venter et al., 1980; Blecher et al., 1981), transferrin receptors (Larrick et al., 1981), and beta-adrenergic (Venter et al., 1980; Fraser et al., 1981) receptors have been shown to recognize sites distant from active ligand binding sites and yet alter ligand binding, while autoantibodies binding to insulin receptors in type B acanthosis nigricans compete directly with insulin binding (Kahn et al., 1976). It is important to emphasize that direct bindings studies with radiolabelled GM-CSF and purified populations of human CFU-MK would be required to directly demonstrate that such mechanisms are occurring in the situation under investigation here.

REFERENCES

Abe T, Fuher P, Bregman MD, Kuramoto A, Murphy MJ Jr. (1988). Factors regulating megakaryocytopoiesis and platelet formation: In Molecular Biology of Hemopoiesis. Ed. by M. Tavassoli, Zanjani ED, Ascensao JL, Abraham NG, Levene AS. Plenum Press, New York, p. 183.

Adams WH, Liu YK, Sullivan LW (1978). Humoral regulation of thrombopoiesis in man. J Lab Clin Med 91:141.

Berridge MV, Fraser JK, Carter JM, Li FK (1988). Effects of recombinant erythropoietin on megakaryocytes and on platelet production in the rat. Blood 72:970.

Blecher M, Bar RS (1981). Receptors and Human Disease. Baltimore, Williams and Wilkins.

Breton-Gorius J, Vainchenker W (1987). Expression of platelet proteins during the in vitro and in vivo differentiation of megakaryocytes and morphological aspects of their maturation. Sem Hematol 23:43.

Brey O, Graner EPR, Wells D (1969). Cyclical thrombocytopenia associated with multiple autoantibodies. Brit Med J 3:397.

Bruno E, Miller ME, Hoffman R (1989). Interacting cytokines regulate in vitro human megakaryocytopoiesis. Blood 76:671.

Bruno E, Briddel R, Hoffman R (1988). Effect of recombinant and purified hematopoietic growth factors on human megakaryocyte colony formation. Exp Hematol 16:371.

Bruno E, Hoffman R (1989). Effect of interleukin-6 on in vitro human megakaryocytopoiesis: its interaction with other cytokines. Exp Hematol. In press.

Clark AC, Kamen R (1987). The human hematopoietic colony stimulating factors. Science 236:1229.

Clark AC, Dessypris EN (1986). Effects of recombinant erythropoietin on murine megakaryocytic colony formation in vitro. J Lab Clin Med 108:423.

Cohen T, Cooney DO (1974). Cyclic thrombocytopenia. Case report and review of literature. Scan J Haemat 12:9.

deAlarcon PA, Schmieder JA, Gringrich R, Klugman MP (1988). Pattern of response of megakaryocytic colony stimulating activity in the serum of patients undergoing bone marrow transplantation. Exp Hematol 16:316.

Dessypris EN, Gleaton JH, Armstrong OL (1987). Effect of human recombinant erythropoietin on human marrow megakaryocyte colony formation in vitro. Br J Haematol 67:265.

Dessypris EN, Gleaton JH, Sawyer ST, Armstrong OL (1987). Suppression of maturation of megakaryocyte colony forming unit in vitro by a platelet-released glycoprotein. J Cell Physiol 130:361.

Donahue RE, Seehra J, Metzger M, LeFebvre D, Rock B, Carbone S, Nathan DG, Garnick M, Sehgal PK, Laston D, LaVallase E, McCoy J, Schendel PF, Norton C, Turner K, Yange YC, Clark SC (1988). Human IL-3 and GM-CSF act synergistically on stimulating hematopoiesis in primates. Science 241:1820.

Donahue RE, Wang EA, Stone DK, Kamen R, Wong GC, Sehgral PK, Nathan DG, Clark SC (1986). Stimulation of hematopoiesis in primates by continuous infusion of recombinant human GM-CSF. Nature 321:872.

Doniach D, Bottazzo GF, Drexhage HA (1982). The autoimmune endocrinopathies. In:Lachman PJ, Peters DK, eds. Clinical aspects of immunology. Vol 2; 4th ed. London:Blackwell, 903.

Drachman DB, Adams RN, Josifek LF, Self SG (1982). Functional activities of autoantibodies to acetylcholine recptors and the clinical severity of myasthenia gravis. N Engl J Med 307:769.

Dukes PP, Egrie JC, Strickland TW, Broure JK, Lin FK (1986). Megakaryocyte colony stimulating activity of recombinant human and monkey erythropoietin, in Evat B, Levine R, Williams N (eds): Megakaryocyte Development and Function. New York, Alan R. Liss, Inc. p.105.

Ebbe S, Stohlman F Jr., Donovan J, Overcash J (1968). Megakaryocytic maturation rate in thrombocytopenic rats. Blood 32:787.

Ebbe S, Yee T, Carpenter D, Phalen E (1988). Megakaryocytes increase in size within ploidy groups in response to the stimulus of thrombocytopenia. Exp Hematol 16:55.

Engstrom K, Lundquist, Soderstrom N (1966). Periodic thrombocytopenia or tidal platelet dysgenesis in a man. Scan J Haematol 3:290.

Eschbach JW, Egrie JC, Downing MR, Browne JK, Adamson JW (1987). Correction of the anemia of end stage renal disease with recombinant human erythropoietin. N Engl J Med 316:73.

Evatt BL, Shreiner DP, Levin J (1974). Thrombopoietic activity of fractions of rabbit plasma: studies in rabbits and mice. J lab Clin Med 83:364.

Fraser CM, Venter JC, Kaliner M (1981). Autonomic abnormalities and autoantibodies to beta-adrenergic receptors. N Engl J Med 305:1165.

Ganser A, Carlo-Stella C, Greher J, Volkers B, Hoelzer D (1987) Effect of recombinant interferons aloha and gamma on human bone marrow derived megakaryocyte progenitor cells. Blood 70:1173.

Ganser H, Lindemann A, Ottman OG, Herrman F, Schulz G, Mertelsmann R, Hoelzer D (1989). Effect of recombinant interleukin-3 in vivo: Aphase I trail. Exp Hematol 17:40.

Geibler K, Hinterberger W, Fisher M, Lechner K (1985). Megakaryocytopoiesis stimulatory factors are highly increased in sera from patients after bone marrow transplantation. Exp Hematol 13:97.

Gewirtz AM, Calabretta B, Rucinshi B, Niewiarowski S, Xu WY (1989). Inhibition of human megakaryocytopoiesis in vitro by platelet factor 4 (PF4) and a synthetic C-terminal PF4 peptide. J Clin Invest, 83:1477.

Granfeld C (1989). Antibody against the insulin receptor causes disappearance of insulin receptors in 3T3 L1 cells: a possible explanation of antibody induced insulin resistance. Proc Natl Acad Sci USA 81:2508.

Harker LA (1968). Kinetics of thrombopoiesis. J Clin Invest 47:458.

Hill R, Levin J (1987). Partial purification of thrombopoietin using lectin chromatography. Exp Hematol 14:752.

Hoffman R, Mazur E, Bruno E, Floyd V (1981). Assay of an activity in the serum of patients with disorders of thrombopoiesis that stimulates formation of megakaryocytic colonies. N Eng J Med 305:533.

Hoffman R, Yang HH, Bruno E, Straneva JE (1985). Purification and partial characterization of a megakaryocyte colony-stimulating factor from human plasma. J Clin Invest 75:1174.

Hoffman R, Briddell RA, vanBesian K, Srour EF, Guscar T, Hudson NW, Ganser A (1989). Acquired cyclic amegakaryocytic thrombocytopenia associated with an immunoglobulin blocking the action of granulocyte-macrophage colony stimulating factor. N Eng J Med 321:97.

Ikebuchi K, Wong GC, Clark SC, Ihle JN, Hirai Y, Ogawa M (1987). Interleukin 6 enhancement of interleukin 3 dependent proliferation of multipotential hematopoietic progenitors.

Ishibashi T, Kimura H, Uchida T, Kariyome S, Friese P, Burstein SA (1989). Recombinant human interleukin 6 (IL-6) directly promotes murine megakaryocyte (MK) maturation. Nouy Re Fr Hematol 31:236.

Ishibashi T, Miller SL, Burstein SA (1987). Type beta transforming growth factor is a potent inhibitor of murine megakaryocytopoiesis in vitro. Blood 69:1737.

Jones JB, Yang TJ, Dale JB, Lange RD (1975). Canine cyclic hematopoiesis: marrow transplantation between liter mates. Bt J Haematol 30:215.

Kahn DCR, Flier JS, Bar RS (1976). The syndrome of insulin resistance and acanthosis migricans: insulin-receptor disorders in man. N Engl J Med 294:739.

Kaushansky K, O'Hara RJ, Berkner K, Segal GM, Hagen FS, Adamson JW (1986). Genomic cloning, characterization and multilineage growth-promoting activity of human granulocyte-macrophage colony-stimulating factor. Proc Natl Acad Sci USA 83:3101.

Kawakita M, Enomoto K, Katayama N, Kishimoto S, Miyake T (1981). Thrombopoiesis and megakaryocyte colony stimulating factors in the urine of patients with idiopathic thrombocytopenic purpura. Br J Haematol 48:609.

Kawakita M, Ogawa M, Goldwasser E, Miyake T (1983). Characterization of human megakaryocyte colony stimulating factor in the urinary extracts from patients with aplastic anemia and idiopathic thrombocytopenic purpura. Blood 61:556.
Kimura H, Burstein SA, Thorning SA, Powell JS, Harker LA, Fialkow PJ, Adamson JW (1984). Human megakaryocytic progenitors (CFU-M) assaying in methylcellulose: physical characteristics and requirements for growth. J Cell Physiol 118:87.
Koeffler HP, Gasson J, Raynud J, Souza L, Shepard M, Munker R (1987). Recombinant human TNF alpha stimulates production of granulocyte colony stimulating factor. Blood 70:55.
Krumwieh D, Seiler FF (1988). Changes of hematopoiesis in cynomolgus monkeys after application of human colony stimulating factors. Exp Hematol 16:551.
Krumwieh D, Seiler FR (1989). In vivo effects of recombinant interleukin-3 alone or in various combination with other cytokines as GM-CSF, G-CSF and Epo in normal cynomolgus monkeys. J Cell Biochem Suppl 132:12,H407.
Larrick JW, Hyman ES (1981). Acquired iron-deficiency caused by an antibody against the transferrin receptor. N Engl J Med 311:214.
Levin J, Evatt BL (1979). Humoral control of thrombopoiesis. Blood Cells 5:105.
Lopez AF, To LD, Yang YC, Gamble JR, Shannon MF, Burns GF, Dyson PG, Juttner CA, Clark S, Vadas MA (1987). Stimulation of proliferation, differentiation and function of human cells by primate interleukin 3. Proc Natl Acad Sci USA 84:2761.
Loughran TP Jr., Clark EA, Price TH, Hammond WP (1986). Adult onset neutropenia is associated with increased large granular lymphocytes. Blood 68:1082.Lu L, Bridell RA, Graham CD, Brandt JE, Bruno E, Hoffman R (1988). Effect of recombinant and purified human hematopoietic growth factors on in vitro colony formation by enriched populations of human megakaryocyte progenitor cells. Br J Haematol 70:149.

Lu L, Briddell RA, Graham CD, Brandt JE, Bruno E, Hoffman R (1988). Effect of recombinant and purified human ahematopoietic growth factors on in vitro colony formation by enriched populations of human megakaryocyte progenitor cells. Br J Maematol 70:149.

Mazur EM, South K (1985). Human megakaryocyte colony-stimulating factor in sera from aplastic dogs: partial purification, characterization and determination of hematopoietic cell lineage specificity. Exp Hematol 13:1164.

Mazur EM, de Alarcon P, South K, Miceli L (1984). Human serum megakaryocyte colony stimulating activity increases in response to intensive cytotoxic chemotherapy. Exp Hematol 12:624.

Mazur EM, Hoffman R, Bruno E (1981). Regulation of human megakaryocytopoiesis. J Clin Invest 68:733.

Mazur EM, Cohen JL, Newton J, Gesner TG, Mufson RA, (1988). Human serum megakaryocyte MK colony stimulating (Meg-CSA) is distinct from interleukin-3 (IL-3), granulocyte macrophage colony stimulating factor (GM-CSF) and phytohemagglutinin stimulated lymphocyte conditioned medium. Blood 72:331a.

Mazur EM, Cohen JE, Wong OG, Clark SC (1987). Modest stimulating effect of recombinant human GM-CSF of colony growth from peripheral blood human megakaryocyte progenitor cells. Exp Hematol 15:1128.

Mazur EM, Hoffman R, Chasis J, Marchesi S, Bruno E (1981). Immunofluorescent identification of human megakaryocyte colonies using an antiplatelet glycoprotein antiserum. Blood 57:277.

Mazur EM, Cohen JL, Bogart L, Mufson RA, Gesner TG, Yang YC, Clark SC (1988). Recombinant globulin interleukin-3 stimulates megakaryocyte colony growth in vitro from human peripheral blood progenitor cells. J Cell Physiol 136:439.

McDonald TP (1988). Thrombopoietin: its biology, purification and characterization. Exp Hematol 16:201.

McDonald TP, Cottrell M, Clift R, Khouri JA, Long MD (1985). Studies on the purification of thrombopoietin from kidney cell culture media. J Lab Clin Med 106:162.

McDonald TP, Cottrell M, Clift RE, Cullen WC, Li FK (1987). High doses of recombinant erythropoietin stimulate platelet production in mice. Exp Hematol 15:719.

McDonald TP, (1988). Current states of thrombopoietin in M. Tavassoli, Zanjani ED, Ascensao JA, Abraham NG, Levine AS (eds): Molecular Biology of Hemopoiesis, Plenum Press p. 243.

McGrath HE, McNiece IK, Clark S, Gillis S, Quesenberry PJ (1989). Interleukin-6 stimulation of murine megakaryocyte colony formation. Clin Res 37:549a.

McNiece IK, McGrath HE, Quesenberry PJ (1988). Granulocyte colony-stimulating factor augments in vitro megakaryocyte colony formation by interleukin-3. Exp Hematol 16:807.

Menitove JE, Pereira J, Hoffman R, Fried W, Cretney C, Aster RH (1987). Cyclic thrombocytopenia attributable to autoantibody directed against the GPIIb/IIIa complex. Blood 70:(Suppl1) 341a.

Menitove JE, Anderson T, Hoffman R, Aster RH (1987). Cyclic autoimmune thrombocytopenia purpura. Blood 62:(Supp 1) 245a.

Messner HA, Jamal N, Izaguirre C (1982). The growth of large megakaryocytic colonies from human bone marrow. J Cell Physiol Suppl 1:45.

Messner HA, Yarnasaki K, Jamal N, Minden MM, Yang YC, Wong GG, Clark SC (1987). Growth of human hemopoietic colonies in response to recombinant gibbon interleukin-3: comparison with human recombinant granulocyte and granulocyte-macrophage colony stimulating factor. Proc Natl Acad Sci USA 84:6765.

Metcalf D (1985). The granulocyte-macrophage colony stimulating factor. Science 229:16.

Mitjavila MT, Vinci G, Villeval JL, Kieffer N, Henri A, Testa U, Breton-Gorius J, Vainchenker W (1988). Human platelet alpha granules contain a non specific inhibition of megakaryocyte colony formation: Its relationship to type B transforming growth factor (TGF-beta). J Cell Physiol 139:93.

Miura M, Jackson CW, Steward SA (1988). Increase in circulating megakaryocyte growth promoting activity (Meg-GPA) following sublethal irradiation is not related to decreased platelets. Exp Hematol 16:139.

Mizoguchi H, Fujiwara Y, Sasaki R, Chiba H (1986). The effect of interleukin-3 and erythropoietin on murine megakaryocyte colony formation in Evatt B, Levine R, Williams N (eds): Megakaryocyte Development and Function. New York, Alan R. Liss Inc., p.111.

Munker R, Gasson J, Ogawa M, Koeffler HP (1986). Recombinant human TNF induces production of granulocyte-macrophage colony stimulating factor. Nature 323:79.

Odell TT Jr., McDonald TP, Detwiter TC (1961). Stimulation of platelet production by serum of platelet depleted rats. Proc Soc Exp Biol Med 108:428.

Pepper H, Leibowitz D, Lindsay S (1956). Cyclical thrombocytopenic purpura related to the menstrual cycle. AMA Arch Pathol 61:1.

Peschel C, Paul WE, O'Hara J, Green I (1987). Effects of B cell stimulatory factor-1/interleukin-4 on hematopoietic progenitor cells. Blood 70:254.

Quesenberry PJ, Ihle JN, McGrath E (1985). The effect of interleukin-3 and GM-CSA-2 on megakaryocyte and myeloid clonal colony formation. Blood 65:214.

Robinson BE, McGrath HE, Quesenberry PJ (1987). Recombinant murine granulocyte macrophage colony stimulating factor has megakaryocyte colony stimulating activity and augments megakaryocyte colony stimulation by interleukin-3. J Clin Invest 79:1648.

Rossi A, Vannucchi AM, Rafanelli D, Ferrini PR (1989). Recombinant human erythropoietin has little influence on megakaryocytopoiesis in mice. Br J Haematol 71:463.

Sakaguchi M, Kawakita M, Matsushita J, Shibuya K, Koishihawa Y, Takatsike (1987). Human erythropoietin stimulates murine megakaryocytopoiesis in serum free culture. Exp Hematol 15:1023.

Sieff CA (1987). Hematopoietic growth factors. J Clin Invest 79:1549.

Sieff CA, Niemeyer CM, Nathan DG, Ekern SC, Bieber FR, Yang Yc, Wong G, Clark SC (1987). Stimulation of human hematopoietic colony formation by recombinant gibbon multi-colony-stimulating factor or interleukin-3. J Clin Invest 80:818.

Sieff CA, Niemeyer CM, Mentzer SJ, Fallen DV (1988). Interleukin 1, tumor necrosis factor and the production of colony-stimulating factors by cultured mesenchymal cells. Blood 72:1316.

Solberg LA Jr., Jamal H, Messner HA (1985). Characterization of human megakaryocytic colony formation in human plasma. J Cell Physiol 124:67.

Solberg LA, Tucker RF, Oles KJ, Mann KG, Moses HL: The effects of type B transforming growth on human hematopoietic cells in vitro. Proceedings of the conference on megakaryocyte development and function. September 18-21, 1985 Woods Hole MA, Abstract p.8.

Sparrow RL, Swee-Huat O, Williams N (1987). Hematopoietic growth factors stimulating murine megakaryocytopoiesis: interleukin-3 is immunologically a distinct form megakaryocyte-potentiator. Leuk Res 10:403.

Spivak JL, Small D, Hollenberg MD (1977). Erythropoietin isolation by affinity chromatography with lectin-agarose derivatives. Proc Natl Acad Sci USA 74:4633.

Straneva JE, Yang HH, Hui SL, Bruno E, Hoffman R (1987). Effects of megakaryocyte colony stimulating factor on terminal cytoplasmic maturation of human megakaryocytes. Exp Hematol 15:657.

Straneva JE, Briddell RA, McDonald TP, Yang HH, Hoffman R (1988). Thrombocytopoiesis stimulating factor (TSF) in aplastic anemia serum accelerates cytoplasmic maturation of human megakaryocytes. Exp Hematol 16:217.

Stroscheck CM, Carpenter G (1989). Down regulation of epidermal growth factor receptors: direct demonstration of receptor degradation in human fibroplasts. J Cell Biol. 98:1048.

Swee-Huat O, Williams N (1986). Biochemical characterization of an in vitro murine megakaryocyte growth activity: megakaryocyte potentiator. Leuk Res 10:403.

Tayrien G, Rosenberg RD (1987). Purification and properties of a megakaryocyte stimulating factor present both in the serum free conditioned medium of human embryonic kidney cells and in thrombocytopenic plasma. J Biol Chem 262:3262.

Teramura M, Katahira J, Hoshino S, Motoji T, Oshimi K, Mizoguchi H (1988). Clonal growth of human megakaryocyte progenitors in serum free cultures: effect of recombinant human interleukin-3. Exp Hematol 16:843.
Tomer A, Schrieber AD, McMillan R, Burstein SA, Cines DB, Thiessen AR, Harker LA (1988). Menstrual cyclic thrombocytopenia. Clin Res 36:615a.
Vainchenker W, Chapman J, Deschamps JF, Vinci G, Bouget J, Titeux M, Breton-Gorius J (1982). Normal human serum contains a factor(s) capable of inhibiting megakaryocyte colony formation. Exp Hematol 10:650.
Vainchenker W, Bouget J, Guichard J, Breton-Gorius J (1974). Megakaryocyte colony formation from human bone marrow precursors. Blood 54:940.
Venter JC, Fraser CM, Harrison LC (1980). Autoantibodies to beta-adrenergic receptors: a possible cause of adrenergic hyporesponsiveness in allergic rhinitis and asthma. science 207:1361.
Wasastjema C (1967). Cyclic thrombocytopenia of acute type. Scand J Haematol 4:380.
Weissman AM, Klausmer RD, Rao K, Harford JB (1986). Exposure of K562 cells to antireceptor monoclonal antibody OKT9 results in rapid redistribution of the enhanced degradation of the transferrin receptor. J Cell Biol 102:951.
Williams N, Eger RR, Jackson HM, Nelson DJ (1982). Two-factor requirement for murine megakaryocyte colony formation. J Cell Physiol 110:101.
Williams N, Jackson H, Iscove NN, Dukes PP, (1984). The role of erythropoietin, thrombopoietic stimulating factor, and myeloid colony-stimulating factors in murine megakaryocyte colony formation. Exp Hematol 12:734.
Williams N, McDonald TP, Rabellino EM (1979). Maturation and regulation of megakaryocytopoiesis. Blood Cells 5:43.
Winerls OG, Pippard MJ, Downing MR, Olwer DO, Reid C, Cotes PM (1986). Effect of human erythropoietin derived from recombinant DNA on the anemia of patients maintained by chronic hemodialysis. Lancet II: 1175.
Wong GC, Witek-Gianott JS, Temple PA, Kriz R, Ferenz C, Hewick RM, Clark SC, Ikebuchi K, Ogawa M (1988). Stimulation of murine hemopoietic colony formation by human IL-6. J Immunol 146:1040.

Wong GC, Clark SC (1988). Multiple actions of interleukin-6 within a cytokine network. Immunol Today 9:137.

Wright DG, Dale DC, Fauci AS, Wolff SM (1981). Human cyclic neutropenia: Clinical review and long term follow up of patients. Medicine 60:1.

Yamasaki K, Solberg LA Jr., Jamal N, Lockwood G, Tritchier D, Curtis JE, Minden MM, Mann KG, Messner HA (1988). Hematopoietic colony growth-promoting activities in the plasma of bone marrow transplant recipients. J Clin Invest 82:255.

Yang HH, Bruno E, Hoffman R (1986). Studies of human megakaryocytopoiesis using an anti-megakaryocyte colony stimulating factor antiserum. J Clin Invest 77:1873.

Yang YC, Tsai S, Wong GG, Clark SC (1988). Interleukin 1 regulation of hematopoietic growth factors by human stomal fibroblasts. J Cell Physiol 134:92.

Young KM, Weiss L (1987). Megakaryocytopoiesis: incorporation of tritiated thymidine by small acetylcholinesterase-positive cells in murine bone marrow during antibody-induced thrombocytopenia. Blood 69:290.

Zucali JR, Dinarello CA, Oblen DJ, Grass MA, Anderson L, Weiner RS (1986). Interleukin 1 stimulates fibroblasts to produce granulocyte-macrophage colony-stimulating activity and prostaglandin E_2. J Clin Invest 78:1316.

Hematopoietic Growth Factors
in Transfusion Medicine, pages 105–112

ERYTHROPOIETIN THERAPY IN AUTOLOGOUS BLOOD DONORS

Lawrence T. Goodnough, M.D.

Associate Professor of Medicine and Pathology
Case Western Reserve University
Cleveland, Ohio 44106

INTRODUCTION

Autologous preoperative blood deposit programs have received widespread support from the medical community because of its potential benefits for patients, blood inventory, and physician transfusion behavior (Wasman, 1987). A previous multicenter study has shown that this practice is underutilized (Toy, 1987); underutilization can be improved with a coordinated program involving hospital blood bank, information services, and physicians (Kruskall, 1986). Nonetheless, we have shown that patients predeposit insufficient autologous blood to minimize or eliminate their subsequent exposure to homologous blood (Goodnough, 1989). Potential problems limiting sufficient autologous blood procurement include: 1) physician underordering; 2) limitations of the storage interval; and 3) erythropoietic response to phlebotomy.

In an analysis of the impact of continuing medical education (CME) on transfusion practice over a 15 month audit interval, homologous blood exposure is reduced in patients who successfully store the amount of autologous blood requested by their physicians, from 12 of 42 (28%) in series 1, to 6/52 (11%) in series 2, and to 1 of 51 (2%) in series 3 (Goodnough, 1989). CME had no impact on the effective storage interval during which blood can be collected and inventoried for elective surgery. Additionally, the percent patients deferred and unable to donate the requested units remained unchanged in each series of patients: 8/50 (16%), 13/65 (20%), and 9/60 (15%) respectively.

We have also shown that homologous blood exposure is not related to physician underordering (11). Fifty-eight patients were asked to donate ≥4 units; 23 (40%) were deferred and 9 of 23 (39%) subsequently received homologous blood. This is compared to 7 of 117 (6%) patients deferred when asked to donate ≤3 units, with 4 of 7 (57%) subsequently receiving homologous blood. We have thus demonstrated that when an autologous predeposit program is accompanied by a CME intervention, homologous blood exposure is related to donor deferral rate rather than physician underordering or inappropriate transfusion behavior. The erythropoietic response to phlebotomy is thus the current limiting factor in procuring sufficient autologous blood to minimize the need for homologous blood exposure. AABB standards have guidelines for elective autologous blood preoperative deposit that include 1) a hemoglobin of no less than 11 g/dl or a packed cell volume of no less than 34%, and 2) phlebotomy no more frequently than every 3 days and not within 72 hours of surgery (Holland, 1987). Recent studies have shown that the endogenous erythropoietin response in autologous donors is not great enough to stimulate compensatory marrow erythropoiesis (Kickler, 1988 and Goodnough, In Press). Such results suggest that supplemental administration of recombinant erythropoietin (rHuEPO) might prevent the development of anemia in these patients and increase the volume of donor blood that can be collected before surgery. To investigate this possibility, we have conducted a randomized, double-blind, placebo-controlled, multicenter study to determine whether rHuEPO can facilitate pre-operative autologous donation.

METHODS

Patients were adults scheduled for elective orthopaedic surgery for which ≥3 units of blood were requested. All study patients were determined to be in good general health (except for the condition for which surgery was scheduled) as evidenced by medical history, physical examination, clinical laboratory tests, and 12 lead electrocardiogram. Patients who exhibited any of the following conditions upon prestudy examination were excluded from admission into the study: history of hematologic disease; history of seizures or uncontrolled hypertension (i.e. diastolic blood pressure of 100 mm Hg or greater); clinically significant ongoing blood loss (e.g.

gastrointestinal), or active inflammatory, infectious or neoplastic diseases which could have compromised the ability to respond to erythropoietin therapy; administration of androgen therapy within 1 month of study entry; administration of cytotoxic agents, immunosuppressives, or other agents known to affect erythropoiesis within 1 month of study entry; history of drug or alcohol abuse within the past 2 years; and blood transfusion or donation of blood within 1 month of study entry.

Female patients could participate if 1) post menopausal for at least one year, or 2) surgically sterile, or 3) taking oral contraceptives for at least one month prior to study entry or agreeing to use barrier and spermacide methods. Female patients of childbearing potential were required to have a negative pregnancy test immediately prior to study entry.

Patients were identified by one of the authors and informed consent obtained. The patients were entered to begin the study medication between 25 and 35 days prior to surgery. Each study patient was scheduled for collection of an autologous unit (450 ml ± 45 ml (15)) twice weekly for 3 weeks (21 days) for a maximum harvest of six units. At each visit, patients received either rHuEPO (600 u/kg) or placebo (diluent) intravenously whether or not blood was actually collected. Patients were deferred from donation if the hematocrit was less than 34%. Each patient took $FeSO_4$, 325 mg orally three times daily during the study interval.

Laboratory tests performed on all study patients initially and at intervals during the study included complete blood counts, stool for occult blood, urinalysis, electrolytes, liver and renal function tests, coagulation studies and iron studies. An enzyme-linked immunosorbent assay (ELISA) performed at Hazleton Biotechnologies Company (Vienna, VA) was used to detect antibodies to recombinant human erythropoietin in serum (Egrie, 1987).

The erythropoietin used in these studies was produced by Amgen Corp. (Thousand Oaks, CA) using recombinant DNA techniques and supplied courtesy of Ortho Pharmaceutical Corporation, Biotech Division (Raritan, NJ). rHuEPO is more than 98 percent pure and is formulated in a sterile, buffered saline and human serum albumin (2.5 mg/ml) solution at 10,000 u/ml. rHuEPO has an amino acid sequence identical to that of human urinary erythropoietin (Lai, 1986); rHuEPO is indistinguishable from human urinary erythropoietin on the basis of all immunological and biological comparisons performed to date. The carbohydrate composition and the immunologic and biologic properties of the natural urinary and recombinant hormones are indistinguishable. The specific activity of the recombinant human erythropoietin was greater than 100,000 units per milligram of hormone (Egrie, 1986).

The exact Wilcoxon midranks test was used to compare the number of units obtained from each group, over both sexes and for each sex. The Wilcoxon rank sum test was used to compare the mean RBC volume on each visit, and the hematocrit (%) on each visit. Fisher's exact test was used to compare the percent deferrals, the number of units meeting the RBC requirement for homologous blood for each group, and the number of patients able to donate 4 or more units in each group. All tests were two-sided and conducted with a 0.05 type 1 error probability.

Fifty-four eligible patients were enrolled and 47 patients completed the study. Five patients removed from study were in the placebo group and two patients removed from study were in the rHuEPO treatment group. There were no differences between the two groups when analyzed for age, sex, surgical procedure, or duration of hospitalization.

RESULTS

Units Collected

Twenty-three patients who were randomized to receive rHuEPO therapy predonated 125 units (5.43 ± 0.2, $m \pm SE$ per patient) compared to 99 units predonated by 24 patients (4.1 ± 0.2, $p<0.05$) who received placebo treatment. The rHuEPO group donated significantly more units than the placebo group when analyzed for males (5.92 ± 0.16 vs 4.56 ± 0.64) and females (4.91 ± 0.6 vs 3.87 ± 0.54), respectively. Over the three week study period, patients treated with rHuEPO were deferred 13 times compared to 45 total deferrals in patients treated with placebo, $p<0.05$.

Only 1/23 (4%) patients treated with rHuEPO were unable to predonate ≥ 4 units, compared to 7/24 (29%) placebo patients ($p<0.05$).

Red Cell Volume Collected

Analysis of RBC volume harvested from patients in each treatment group is shown in Table I:

TABLE I

RED BLOOD CELL (RBC) VOLUME PROCURRED

(ALL PATIENTS)

Donation	1		2		3		4		5		6		
Placebo (n)*	24		24		23		17		8		3		
($\bar{x}$)**	183		168		156		156		161		158		
% Patients donating	100		100		96		71		33		12		
RBC Volume ***	183	+	168	+	149	+	110	+	54	+	20	=	684
EPO (n)*	23		23		23		22		19		15		
($\bar{x}$)**	188		177		172		173		173		177		
% Patients donating	100		100		100		91		83		65		
RBC Volume ***	188	+	177	+	172	+	166	+	144	+	115	=	962

* Number of Blood Units Donated
** Mean RBC Volume (ml) Per Unit
***Average RBC Volume (ml) Procurred in Each Group

The RBC volume collected from each patient was determined by multiplying the blood unit volume (450 ml) x the donation Hct (%). Mean RBC volume per autologous blood unit collected was significantly higher in the rHuEPO group (174 ml) compared to placebo group at the third and fourth donations (156 ml) ($p<0.05$). Analysis of the RBC volume by unit showed that 23/98 (24%) placebo units had <154 ml RBC (AABB minimum standards for homologous blood units (15)) compared to 15/122 (12%) rHuEPO units, $p<0.05$. Patients treated with rHuEPO donated 41% more total RBC volume per donor than donors treated with placebo (961 vs 683 ml, $p<0.05$). This difference is also shown when analyzed be sex; males treated with rHuEPO donated 42% more RBC volume (1097 vs 776 ml) than placebo males and rHuEPO females donated 29% more RBC volume (809 vs 627 ml) than placebo females.

Hematocrit (%) data for males and females in both treatment groups was analyzed. Significant differences ($p<0.05$) between the two groups were demonstrable from the third visit (7.2 ± 0.8 days, m ± SEM) until the end of study. Patients receiving rHuEPO had significantly less hematocrit decline (-5.5 vs -8.8%, $p<0.05$) and higher surgical admission hematocrit (38.6% vs 35.2%, $p<0.05$) than did patients receiving placebo. Significantly lower admission and discharge hematocrits were seen in the placebo group (35.2% and 30.5%, respectively) compared to the rHuEPO group (38.6% and 33.5%, respectively), $p < 0.05$. rHuEPO patients received 89 of 122 (73%) units donated compared to 73 of 98 (74%) units donated by the placebo group. One rHuEPO-treated patient subsequently received 2 homologous blood (HB) units compared to two placebo-treated patients (3 and 2 HB units; respectively).

No differences were seen in patient incidence of adverse events between treatment groups. Recorded systolic and diastolic blood pressures were no different between treatment groups throughout the study interval. Patient #0501 (placebo group) suffered a myocardial infarction after donating three blood units over 12 days. This patient had no previous history of cardiac disease and had a hematocrit of 37% determined before the time of infarction. Patient #0305 developed a peripheral artery thrombosis with a hematocrit of 40.9% after predonating two blood units over 8 days. This patient was not known to have significant peripheral vascular disease at admission and had been placed on β-blocker medication for treatment of hypertension. However, subsequent investigation indicated a history of arteriosclerosis.

Radioimmunoassay for the detection of erythropoietin antibody was performed pre-study, post-study, and 1 month post-study on 45/47 patients. All assays were negative for the detection of antibody, including the 41 of 47 patients tested 1 month post-study.

DISCUSSION

This study has demonstrated the ability of rHuEPO to facilitate autologous blood donation. Patients treated with rHuEPO donated 41% more RBC volume per patient over the study interval than did patients treated with placebo (961 vs 683 ml, respectively). The efficacy of rHuEPO to facilitate autologous RBC donation was seen for both males and females (42% and 29% increase respectively). In males, the rHuEPO effect was seen in an increased Hct (%) as well as number of units successfully donated (71 of 72 (99%) possible units compared to 41 of 54 (76%) possible units in the placebo group). Similarly in females, the rHuEPO effect was seen in the number of units successfully donated (54 of 66 (82%) possible units compared to 58 of 90 (64%) possible units in the placebo group) as well as an increased Hct (%). In our previous study of 175 consecutive autologous donors scheduled for elective orthopaedic surgery we have previously shown that 23/58 (40%) of patients are unable to donate $\geq$ 4 units (Goodnough, 1988). Results of our current study confirm that when patients are enrolled in an autologous program designed to procure up to 6 units of blood in 3 weeks, 7/24 (29%) of placebo-treated patients are unable to donate $\geq$ 4 AB units while only 1/23 (4%) rHuEPO-treated patients were unable to store $\geq$ 4 units ($p<0.05$). While a longer donation interval may allow the larger collection of more units of autologous blood, our previous study has demonstrated that the effective donation interval for orthopaedic procedures is no different before educating the physician staff (21.6 ± 1.3 days) than afterward (22.6 ± 1.3 days) (Goodnough, 1989). A previous aggressive phlebotomy study has been performed in baboons (Levine, 1988). The baboon phlebotomy schedule did not conform to AABB standards for human autologous donation (Holland, 1987): a blood unit was drawn any day the hematocrit was greater than 30% and iron supplementation was given intravenously. The dose of rHuEPO given was 750 u/kg, compared to 600 u/kg in our study. Nevertheless, this previous study was also a randomized, placebo controlled trial (n=6 in each arm) in which rHuEPO-treated baboons donated 35% more blood than controls. The results of our present study indicate that these results can be achieved in humans given oral iron therapy who follow an autologous blood donation program according to AABB standards.

REFERENCES

Egrie JC, Cotes PM, Lane J, et al (1987). Development of radioimmunoassays for human erythropoietin using recombinant erythropoietin as tracer and immunogen. J. Immunol. Methods 99:235-241.

Egrie JC, Strickland TW, Lane J, et al (1986). Characterization and biologic effects of recombinant human erythropoietin. Immunobiology 172:213-24.

Goodnough LT (1988). Autologous blood. JAMA 259:2405.

Goodnough LT and Brittenham G (1988). Limitations of the erythropoietic response to serial phlebotomy: Implications for autologous blood donor programs. J Lab Clin Med, In Press.

Goodnough LT, Wasman J, Corlucci K, Chernosky A (1989). Limitations to donating adequate autologous blood prior to elective orthopaedic surgery. Arch Surgery 124:494-496.

Holland PV, Schmidt PJ (eds): Standards for blood banks and transfusion services, 12th edition, Arlington, VA. American Association of Blood Banks, 1987, p 39.

Kickler TS, Spivak JL (1988). Effect of repeated whole blood donations on serum immunoreactive erythropoietin levels in autologous donors. JAMA 260:65-67.

Kruskall MS, Glazer EE, Leonard SS, Willson SC, Pacinin DG, Donovan LM, Ransil BJ (1986). Utilization and effectiveness of a hospital autologous preoperative blood donor program. Transfusion 26:335-340.

Lai P-H, Everett R, Wang FF, Arakawat, Goldwasser E, (1986). The primary structure of human erythropoietin. J Biol Chem 261:3116-21.

Levine EA, Rosen AL, Gould SA, et al (1988). Recombinant human erythropoietin and autologous blood donation. Surgery 104:365-369.

Toy PT, Strauss RG, Stehling LC, et al (1987). Predeposit autologous blood for elective surgery: A multicenter study. N Engl J Med 316:517-520.

Wasman J, Goodnough LT (1987). Effect of autologous blood donation for elective surgery on physician transfusion behavior: a matched control study. JAMA 258:3135-3137.

Hematopoietic Growth Factors
in Transfusion Medicine, pages 113–120

ERYTHROPOIETIN THERAPY IN AIDS

David H. Henry, MD

Department of Medicine, University
of Pennsylvania School of Medicine,
Graduate Hospital, Philadelphia,
Pennsylvania 19146

INTRODUCTION

Anemia is common in patients with HIV infection and is increasingly common with disease progression. Asymptomatic, HIV antibody positive patients have a 10% incidence of anemia while AIDS-related complex (ARC) patients have a 50% incidence and AIDS patients have a 75% incidence.

The anemia is often severe enough to require transfusion. At the Graduate Hospital (350 beds) in Philadelphia, approximately 30 units of packed red cells are transfused in hospitalized AIDS patients each month while an equal number of units are transfused in outpatients for a total of 60 units a month. At a cost of $250 per unit for preparation, not including the indirect costs of administering a transfusion and treating any side effects, AIDS-related transfusions cost $180,000 per year in just one moderate sized hospital. The need for transfusion will only increase in the future since the Centers for Disease Control currently estimates 1-2 million Americans are HIV infected and projects there will be 300,000 cases of AIDS in the United States by 1991.

Transfusion is not only expensive in terms of dollars and resources, but also may actually be harmful to the immune system. There is adequate evidence in the oncology literature detailing both a decreased time to recurrence and decreased overall survival in some transfused cancer patients (Wu and Little, 1988). Natural killer cells and CD4 lymphocytes fall and CD8 lymphocytes rise in heavily transfused patients (Perkins, 1989). This may translate into an adverse effect in AIDS patients, but this issue remains to be studied.

This section of the monograph will examine three issues in AIDS patients who are anemic: 1) Why do AIDS patients develop anemia, 2) What is the relationship of the endogenous erythropoietin level in AIDS patients to the anemia and 3) Is there a role for the administration of exogenous erythropoietin in the anemia of AIDS.

ANEMIA AND AIDS

All three classical mechanisms of anemia can contribute to the anemia of AIDS, namely, decreased bone marrow production, increased peripheral destruction, and blood loss. Decrease in bone marrow production is the most important of the three and can occur for several reasons. The HIV virus itself is responsible for the anemia, in part. One study has demonstrated that the earliest committed red cell precursors continue to grow normally in culture when infected with the HIV virus, but their proliferation is markedly suppressed when grown in the presence of HIV antibody positive serum (Donahue et al., 1987). Presumably, HIV related antigens are expressed on the surface of infected cells and then recognized by the antibody in HIV positive serum.

HIV infection also causes a marked alteration in the cytokine environment necessary for normal marrow function. For example, levels of gamma interferon are reduced and monocyte derived suppressor substances are increased (Laurence et al., 1983; Murray et al., 1984). Specific growth factors necessary for erythropoiesis are also reduced; erythropoietin levels are virtually always lower than would be expected for any given degree of anemia. This phenomenon may not be special to the HIV infection; but rather, simply a part of the anemia of chronic disease (ACD) which all HIV infected patients have by definition. Other infections are also common in the bone marrow. Tuberculosis and Mycobacterium avium-intracellulare can be stained and cultured from some marrows. Fungal infections include Coccidioidomycosis, Cryptococcus, and Histoplasmosis; and both CMV and HSV have been grown out of the bone marrow in AIDS patients.

Many medications suppress bone marrow function and these include antibiotics, particularly those with a sulfa moiety, and Azidothymidine (AZT) which can be a particularly potent inhibitor of bone marrow function. AZT is a thymidine analog and inhibits the reverse transcriptase enzyme of HIV; but it also inhibits normal cellular DNA polymerases, particularly in the bone marrow, which probably accounts for its increased bone marrow toxicity.

Finally, B12 levels are lower than normal in as many as 30% of AIDS patients probably because of a gastropathy. When present, this B12 deficiency may contribute to the development of anemia (Herbert, 1988).

A striking variety of abnormal bone marrow histologies have been observed. A recent review on this subject noted that the marrow cellularity was usually normal or increased, but that erythroid precursors were decreased and frequently dysplastic. Myeloid dysplasia and plasmacytosis were common. Megakaryocytes were either adequate or increased. Marrow iron stores were usually adequate or increased, and lymphoid aggregates were occasionally present. There was also a tendency toward increased reticulin formation which may account for as many as 1/3 of bone marrow examinations being dry taps in AIDS patients (Zon and Groopman, 1988).

Another possible mechanism of anemia is increased peripheral destruction of red cells. While it is not unusual to find a positive Coomb's test, either direct or indirect, it is very unusual to find an autoimmune hemolytic anemia. It is also possible that a non-immune hemolytic anemia contributes to the anemia in some AIDS patients, especially those on AZT. It is not unusual to see an abrupt decrease in hemoglobin of as much as 50% in an occasional patient taking AZT. This cannot be attributed to bone marrow suppression alone, but must be due to a shortened red cell survival as well. The mechanism of this presumed AZT-associated hemolysis is unknown.

Finally, blood loss itself may contribute to AIDS-related anemia. In a hospitalized patient population, phlebotomy is not insignificant. Also, thrombocytopenia can occur and lead to significant bleeding. In the early stages of the disease, immune thrombocytopenia is most often the mechanism; while late in the disease, bone marrow failure is more likely the etiology of thrombocytopenia.

ERYTHROPOIETIN LEVELS AND THE ANEMIA OF AIDS

Erythropoietin is a glycoprotein hormone that directs

the development and maintenance of the red cell mass. If normal human volunteers are maintained on iron but made anemic by repeated phlebotomy, erythropoietin levels (normal 4-26 mU/ml) begin to increase rapidly at a hematocrit below approximately 35 (Kickler and Spivak, 1988). If, however, iron deficiency is allowed to occur, the rate of erythropoietin rise is much steeper. Conversely, as the hematocrit falls in patients with a chronic inflammatory process such as infection or cancer, the rate of rise is much flatter and "inappropriately low" for any given degree of anemia. This flatter erythropoietin response to anemia is typical of the anemia of chronic disease (ACD) which has three characteristic features: a slight shortening of red cell survival, hypoferremia with decreased iron reutilization but increased iron stores, and a decreased erythropoietin response to any level of anemia (Lee, 1983).

To determine how significant the inadequate endogenous erythropoietin levels were in ACD, Means, et al, gave exogenous erythropoietin to two patients with rheumatoid arthritis and ACD. Both patients had an increase in hemoglobin, demonstrating that the poor iron reutilization can be overcome if sufficient erythropoietin stimulation to erythropoiesis is given (Means et al., 1989).

By definition, patients with AIDS have ACD by virtue of their chronic infection with HIV. They uniformly demonstrate a failure to generate appropriate levels of erythropoietin for any degree of anemia. However, if AZT is given, a striking elevation of erythropoietin can occur in some patients who still continue to be anemic (Spivak et al., 1989). The reason for this marked elevation in some patients is not clear but may suggest more than one mechanism for AZT-induced marrow toxicity.

rHuEPO IN THE ANEMIA OF AIDS

Based on these observations, a double-blind, randomized multi-center trial was initiated in anemic AIDS patients taking AZT (Rudnick et al., 1989). This trial used the genetically engineered form of erythropoietin called recombinant human erythropoietin (rHuEPO). rHuEPO was first cloned in 1985 and is now produced in Chinese hamster ovary cells in culture. It is biochemically, immunologically, and physiologically identical to human urinary erythropoietin. Patients were given either rHuEPO at a dose of 100 units/kilogram or placebo IV three times per week for either

12 weeks or until a target hematocrit of 38-40% was achieved. The objectives of the study were to examine the safety of rHuEPO, its efficacy regarding transfusion requirement and hemoglobin, and quality of life.

Sixty-three patients entered the trial and the results are shown in Tables 1 and 2. Table 1 illustrates the change in transfusion requirement during the study. The results are displayed as average number of units transfused per patient per month at the beginning and at the end of the study. When all patients were analyzed, there was no difference between those who received rHuEPO versus placebo. However, retrospectively, a cutoff level for erythropoietin of 500 mU/ml was found to differentiate a "low" erythropoietin group (≤500 mU/ml) from a high erythropoietin group (>500 mU/ml). When these two subsets were analyzed, a significant decrease in transfusion requirement was demonstrated in the low erythropoietin group in favor of those patients receiving rHuEPO. There was no such difference demonstrated in the high erythropoietin group between rHuEPO or placebo treated patients.

TABLE 1. Average Number of Units of Blood Transfused per Patient per Month

Group	N	Baseline	Study End
<u>All Patients</u>			
rHuEPO	29	1.74	1.48
Placebo	34	1.87	2.58
<u>Low EPO Level</u> (≤500 mU/ml)			
rHuEPO	22	1.31	0.84*
Placebo	26**	1.68	2.74
<u>High EPO Level</u> (>500 mU/ml)			
rHuEPO	7	3.10	3.50
Placebo	6**	3.32	2.78

*p<0.05
**EPO value not available for 1 patient in this group

Table 2 displays the number of patients who were

transfusion dependent at the beginning of the study and at the end. Here, also, there was no significant difference when all patients were analyzed, but a significant difference was again demonstrated when patients were separated into the same low and high baseline endogenous erythropoietin groups. In the low erythropoietin group only, there was a significant reduction in the number of patients who were transfusion dependent at the end of the study compared to the beginning in favor of the rHuEPO treated group.

TABLE 2. Number of Patients Transfused per Month

Group	N	Baseline	Study End
<u>All Patients</u>			
rHuEPO	29	23	11
Placebo	34	27	21
<u>Low EPO Level</u> (≤500 mU/ml)			
rHuEPO	22	16	5*
Placebo	26**	21	17
<u>High EPO Level</u> (>500 mU/ml)			
rHuEPO	7	7	6
Placebo	6**	6	4

*p<0.05
**EPO value not available for 1 patient in this group

In order for the results in Tables 1 and 2 to be meaningful, an analysis of the average AZT dosage between rHuEPO treated and placebo treated groups was performed. A significant change in AZT dose in one group versus the other could have accounted for the study transfusion results. As is commonly observed with AZT, there was a tendency for AZT dosage to decrease in all patients in all groups over time, but there were no between group differences in any patient subset at any time. Therefore, there was no significant difference in AZT dosage that could account for the results of the study.

Side effects attributable to rHuEPO were remarkably

uncommon. Fever, fatigue, weakness, rash, headache, and diarrhea are common in AIDS patients; but there were no significant differences in their frequency between rHuEPO and placebo treated groups. Therefore, the symptoms observed could be attributed to the underlying disease process as opposed to any significant increase in adverse effect from the rHuEPO itself.

A visual analog questionnaire was administered to all patients at the beginning, middle, and end of the study to try to assess quality of life changes. While there was no significant difference noted between rHuEPO and placebo treated groups, there was a trend in favor of improvement in energy level and improvement in quality of life in the low erythropoietin group treated with rHuEPO.

In summary, HIV-related anemia is quite common, and increasingly so as the disease progresses. Its etiology is multifactorial, but bone marrow underproduction is the main mechanism. AZT may increase the degree of anemia, and transfusion is frequently required for palliation of symptoms. Baseline endogenous erythropoietin levels are generally low in AIDS patients, but may be quite high in some patients taking AZT. rHuEPO can be safely administered to AIDS patients. At the rHuEPO doses used in this study, anemic AIDS patients taking AZT with baseline erythropoietin levels less than 500 mU/ml had a significant reduction in transfusion requirement and an improvement in overall quality of life. Further studies are underway to examine whether higher doses of rHuEPO can overcome the anemia in patients with higher baseline endogenous erythropoietin levels.

REFERENCES

Donahue RE, Johnson MM, Zon LI, Clark SC, Groopman JE (1987). Suppression of *in vitro* haematopoiesis following human immunodeficiency virus infection. Nature 326:200-203.

Herbert V (1988). B12 deficiency in AIDS. JAMA 260(19):2837.

Kickler TS, Spivak JL (1988). Effect of repeated whole blood donations on serum immunoreactive erythropoietin levels in autologous donors. JAMA 260(2):65-67.

Laurence J, Gottlieb AB, Kunkel HG (1983). Soluble

suppressor factors in patients with acquired immune deficiency syndrome and its prodrome. Elaboration *in vitro* by T lymphocyte-adherent cell interactions. J. Clin Invest 72:2072-2081.

Lee GR (1983). The anemia of chronic disease. Semin Hematol 20:61-80.

Means RT, Olsen NJ, Krantz SB, Dessypris EN, Graber SE, Stone WJ, O'Neil VL, Pincus T (1989). Treatment of the anemia of rheumatoid arthritis with recombinant human erythropoietin: Clinical and *in vitro* studies. Arthritis and Rheumatism 32:1-5.

Murray HW, Rubin BY, Masur H, Roberts RB (1984). Impaired production of lymphokines and immune (gamma) interferon in the acquired immunodeficiency syndrome. N Engl J Med 310:883-889.

Perkins HA (1989). Transfusion-Induced Immunologic Unresponsiveness. Transfusion Medicine Reviews 2(4):196-203.

Rudnick SA, Erythropoietin Study Group (1989). Human Recombinant (r-HuEPO): a double-blind, placebo-controlled study in acquired immunodeficiency syndrome (AIDS) patients with anemia induced by disease and AZT. J Clin Oncol 8:2(abstract).

Spivak JL, Barnes DC, Fuchs E, Quinn TC (1989). Serum Immunoreactive Erythropoietin in HIV-infected patients. JAMA 261:3104-3107.

Wu H, Little AG (1988). Perioperative Blood Transfusions and Cancer Recurrence. J Clin Oncol 6:1348-1354.

Zon LI, Groopman JE (1988). Hematologic manifestations of the human immune deficiency virus (HIV). Semin Hematol 25:208-218.

Hematopoietic Growth Factors
in Transfusion Medicine, pages 121–128

THE USE OF RECOMBINANT HUMAN GRANULOCYTE-MACROPHAGE COLONY-STIMULATING FACTOR IN AUTOLOGOUS BONE MARROW TRANSPLANTATION

William P. Peters, M.D., Ph.D., Joanne Kurtzberg, M.D., Susan Atwater, M.D., Michael Borowitz, M.D., Ph.D., Murali Rao, M.D., Mark Currie, M.D., Colleen Gilbert, RPh, Elizabeth J. Shpall, M.D., Roy B. Jones, M.D., Ph.D., Maureen Ross, M.D. Ph.D

From the Duke University Bone Marrow Transplant Program, Departments of Medicine, Pathology, Pediatrics, Radiology.

INTRODUCTION

Extensive *in vitro* experiments have revealed that hematopoiesis in man is under the control of a series of glycoproteins which work in a concerted manner to regulate bone marrow proliferation and the composition of the cellular elements in the blood. In the last five years, the application of molecular techniques to this problem has led to the identification, cloning, *in vitro* expression, and formulation for clinical use of a series of the colony-stimulating factors for trials in various myelosuppressed states. At least eleven colony-stimulating factors have been identified, and at least five different products (G-CSF, GM-CSF, M-CSF, IL-3, and IL-1) have entered clinical evaluation. Thus far, the clinical experience appears to mimic closely the effects predicted from *in vitro* and preclinical studies.

Characteristics of the Colony-Stimulating Factors

The colony-stimulating factors represent a group of natural glycoproteins, range in molecular weight from 18 to above 90,000 daltons. All appear to be glycosylated in their native states, although the degree of glycosylation is variable, with G-CSF having minimal glycosylation, and others, such as GM-CSF, having variable as well as significant amounts of glycosylation. The precise importance of glycosylation in the functioning of these molecules is unclear. In certain settings, such as erythropoietin, removal of the carbohydrate residue results in the substantial reduction of the therapeutic activity of the compound. In others, for example, granulocyte macrophage colony-stimulating factor (GM-CSF), removal of the carbohydrate from the protein results in an increase of the binding coefficients of the molecule to its receptor, and an increase in the specific activity of the molecule. The importance of these changes in the clinical setting is unclear. Direct comparisons among various products produced either *E. coli*, and therefore non-glycosylated, or yeast or Chinese hamster ovary cells (CHO), have not been performed and would be important for final resolution of differences in therapeutic and toxic effects related to these molecules.

The colony-stimulating factors, in general, appear to be able to enhance the capacity of progenitor cells and their progeny for proliferation, and are as well necessary for survival of the progenitor, and in some instances, important for differentiation. While lineage specificity is suggested by the nomenclature for these molecules -- for example, granulocyte macrophage colony-stimulating factor -- this restriction, does not necessarily hold. Granulocyte macrophage colony-stimulating factor, for example, will stimulate the formation not only of granulocyte and macrophage colonies *in vitro*, but also proliferation and differentiation of erythroid and multipotential progenitors. In addition, these molecules have a broad spectrum of activities on progenitors, as well as on mature cells. GM-CSF will shorten the delay in onset of proliferation, shorten the mean cycle time, and will initiate and sustain the hematopoietic precursor through a complete cycle resulting in cell division. Actions now attributed to GM-CSF's include enhancement of eosinophil killing activity, enhancement of oxidative response of neutrophils, enhancement of ADCC, inhibition of neutrophil migration, enhancement of phagocytosis and chemotaxis, as well as hydrogen peroxide production. It is important to note that these effects may be dose-dependent, and the effects on functional enhancement may occur at doses different from those on proliferation, a feature that may be of importance clinically.

The duration of exposure to the CSF may, as well, play an important role in its modulation of biological activities. Short-term exposure of mature granulocytes to GM-CSF increases the number and affinity of the chemotactic peptide receptors by approximately three-fold, and will enhance neutrophil chemotaxis by about 85%. On the other hand, exposure of neutrophils to longer periods of time converts high-affinity GM-CSF receptors to low affinity receptors, and as well enhances neutrophil oxidative metabolism. At this stage, the enhanced chemotaxic activity noted after brief exposure is no longer evident. Marked changes in the antigenic phenotypes of cells will also be noted. GM-CSF will induce a rapid increase in the expression of the CR3 (the receptor for 3CB) on the granulocyte and monocyte cell surface. This receptor which is detected by the monoclonal antibody MO1 is one of a family of surface glycoproteins associated with adhesion which have differing alpha and common beta subunits. Upon exposure to GM-CSF, CR3 is translocated to the plasma membrane, resulting in a 5- to 10-fold increase in the binding of anti-MO1 binding. The rapidity of induction of MO1 is consistent with the observation that gelatinase-containing organelles are a source of this intracellular CR3 pool.

Potential for CSF's in Intensive Chemotherapy Programs.

The major morbidity associated with chemotherapy is infections and bleeding. In our program, 40% of treatment-related mortality is directly attributable to bacterial or fungal infections. It was demonstrated in the 1960's by Bodie and his colleagues that the duration and severity of neutropenia correlates with the percentage of serious infections encountered by patients. Hence, utilization of strategies resulting in the reduction of the period of time of severe myelsuppression can be expected to reduce the morbidity and mortality of high-dose therapy. Since there is abundant experimental and clinical data that dose intensification is associated with improved therapeutic results in the treatment of various malignant diseases, the potential to reduce the morbidity and to permit dose intensification has profound implications for improvement of therapeutic responses in the treatment of malignant disease. The molecular cloning, *in vitro* expression and formulation of the colony-stimulating factors offer the potential to explore these therapeutic options in man.

It may well be that the importance of the CSF's extend beyond the improvement in infectious complications. Examination of the average toxicity of patients who remain myelosuppressed in the Bone Marrow Transplant Program indicate that with increasing durations of myelosuppression, there is an increase in the overall average toxicity that is seen in patients. Hence, the longer a patient remains myelosuppressed, the more likely that hepatic, renal, pulmonary or other toxicities are likely to occur. This is not surprising given the fact that continued myelosuppression renders the patient susceptible to further infections, requires the continued use of antibiotics and antifungals, and in general the utilization of additional medications. Coupled with the effects of intensive therapy itself, extended periods of myelosuppression will yield increased organ system injury. Thus, the ability to reduce the period of myelosuppression can be expected to be associated with a reduction in overall toxicity.

The hematologic reconstitution following high dose CPA/cDDP/BCNU and autologous bone marrow support is very typical and lends itself to an evaluation of the impact of a systemically infused growth factor on hematopoietic recovery and function. Our previous studies have demonstrated that the time to recovery of a WBC > $1000/mm^3$ is 17.4 $\pm$ 2.7 days. Our current trials with human recombinant granulocyte macrophage colony stimulating factor (rHuGM-CSF) provide an opportunity to study hematopoiesis in rHuGM-CSF treated patients and controls to (1) delineate the "normal" pattern of hematopoietic reconstitution after ABMT, (2) to determine the toxicity of rHuGM-CSF when administered in the setting of high dose combination chemotherapy and autologous marrow transplantation, and (3) to determine the effects of rHuGM-CSF on the functional capacity of bone marrow and granulocytes maturing during rHuGM-CSF administration.

METHODS

Patient Population

Forty eight patients with histologically confirmed breast cancer or melanoma were studied during phase I and II trials of rHuGM-CSF administration. The details of patient selection, pretreatment characteristics and experimental design are or will be provided elsewhere[1] . All twenty-four prior consecutive patients treated with an identical high-dose combination chemotherapy regimen from January 1985 to December 1986 served as a control population for comparison; ten additional contemporaneous patients treated with the same chemotherapy program but not receiving rHuGM-CSF had evaluation of granulocyte function.

Administration of Chemotherapy and rHuGM-CSF

All patients studied received the same chemotherapy program which consisted of cyclophosphamide (1875 mg/m^2, days -6, -5, -4), cisplatin (165 mg/m^2 as a 72 hour continuous intravenous infusion days -6 to -3), and carmustine (600 mg/m^2; day-3). Recombinant HuGM-CSF was begun three hours after infusion of autologous bone marrow at the end of day 0. Bone marrow aspiration and biopsy was performed prior to therapy and at five day intervals following bone marrow autografting. The production and preparation of rHuGM-CSF is described elsewhere[34]. Briefly, complementary DNA encoding human GM-CSF was cloned and expressed by Genetics Institute, Inc. (Cambridge, Mass.), and rHuGM-CSF was formulated as a lyophilized powder by Sandoz Pharmaceuticals (Basel, Switzerland). It was reconstituted in sterile water and added to 500 ml of 5% dextrose with 0.45% saline before administration. Nineteen patients received rHuGM-CSF by continuous intravenous infusion for 14 days at doses ranging from 1.2 to 19.2 mcg/kg/day of aglycosylated rHuGM-CSF protein; twelve patients received 21 day continuous infusions of either 4.8 (five patients) or 9.6 mcg/kg/day (seven patients) aglycosylated rHuGM-CSF infusion; fifteen patients received 4.8 mcg/kg/day (eight patients), 9.6 mcg/kg/day (eight patients) or 19.2 mcg/kg/day aglycosylated rHuGM-CSF as a daily four hour infusion for a planned 21 days. The use of rHuGM-CSF as described was approved by the Duke University Institutional Review Board.

RESULTS

Toxicity

The use of rHuGM-CSF was in general well tolerated. When used as a continuous infusion at doses from 1.2 to 9.6 mcg/kg/day, protein by amino acid analysis, side effects were not dose-limiting and included dependant myalgias, rash, hypotension, fever[2], weight gain, and pleural and pericardial effusions. With the exception of the dependent myalgias, fever, weight gain and hypotension, the frequency of these side effects was not clearly different from other patients not receiving rHuGM-CSF. At 9.6 - 19.2 mcg/kg/day of continuous infusion rHuGM-CSF 10/22 (45%) of patients developed hypotension (MAP < 70). Of these 10 patients, 80% had pleural effusions and peripheral edema. The hypotension began between days 7-10 (8/10 patients). The development of hypotension correlated with serum TNF elevation. Measurement of total blood volume by radiolabeled I^{125} albumin showed an increase during rHuGM-CSF infusion from 4607 $\pm$ 912 to 6223 ml $\pm$ 950. Cardiac evaluation by MUGA or ECHO of 4 patients showed normal left ventricular function. Swan-Ganz monitoring in two hypotensive, but non-septic patients showed an increased cardiac index and a low systemic vascular resistance index with a normal pulmonary artery occlusion pressure[3].

Despite the appearance of toxicity related to rHuGM-CSF at high doses, the administration of rHuGM-CSF was associated with reduced clinical morbidity during the GM-CSF administration. During the administration of rHuGM-CSF, there was objective evidence of clinical benefit with a reduced bacteremia rate, reduced treatment related mortality, and reduced hepatic and renal dysfunction compared to historical controls[34].

Effects of rHuGM-CSF on Bone Marrow Morphology

Serial analysis of bone marrow biopsies from patients receiving rHuGM-CSF demonstrated that by the end of the infusion, 65% of patients had a bone marrow cellularity of greater than 20%[34]. There was considerable variation in the response of individual patients although in the aggregate, the patients receiving rHuGM-CSF had a greater cellularity than a series of contemporaneous controls[4]. This result will require confirmation by a prospective, comparative trial.

Effects of rHuGM-CSF on Circulating Counts

Patients receiving rHuGM-CSF showed a dose dependent increase in circulating leukocytes at the end of the infusion compared to historical controls [5]. The pattern of peripheral leukocyte recovery after a 14-day continuous intravenous infusion of rHuGM-CSF was remarkable for four features: (1) the first appearance of leukocytes on peripheral smear did not differ significantly from the historical control population; (2) once cells began to appear (after 8-10 days from marrow infusion) there was an acceleration of the rate of leukocyte recovery compared to historical controls reaching an equivalent peripheral leukocyte count 10 days earlier at the end of the CSF infusion compared to that observed in control patients; (3) a rapid fall in leukocyte counts following discontinuation of the rHuGM-CSF; and (4) hematopoietic recovery following discontinuation of rHuGM-CSF proceeding in a manner comparable to controls.

Effects of rHuGM-CSF on Granulocyte Margination and Migration

The administration of rHuGM-CSF results in elevated peripheral leukocyte and granulocyte counts. However, cessation of continuous rHuGM-CSF infusion resulted in a rapid decline in peripheral leukocyte counts in normal non-human primates[6], patients with the acquired immunodeficiency syndrome[7] and myelodysplasia[8], and in the autologous bone marrow transplantation setting in both non-human primates[9] and man. The rapidity of the fall in peripheral granulocytes suggests that mechanisms other than production may be operative. Effects of rHuGM-CSF on leukocyte margination or migration might contribute to rapid changes in the peripheral leukocyte counts. Further, rHuGM-CSF has been demonstrated to be identical to neutrophil migration inhibition factor (NIF-T)[10]. This inhibitory effect on neutrophil migration may have important clinical implications where granulocyte mobility is relevant for host defense. Alternatively, the ability of GM-CSF to enhance macrophage function may be able to compensate for this defect in migration, or because the severely infected state is not mimicked by this model, significant clinical infections may be handled differently.

To analyze the effect of rHuGM-CSF on leukocyte margination, we labelled purified autologous granulocytes with ^{111}-Indium and administered these labelled granulocytes to four patients with metastatic breast cancer or melanoma receiving high dose alkylating agent chemotherapy and autologous bone marrow support. Patients were studied before initiation of chemotherapy and again after 14-21 days of continuous intravenous rHuGM-CSF infusion at a time when peripheral blood counts were similar. Epinephrine (0.3 mg sc) was administered to produce temporary leukocyte demargination and the marginating granulocyte fraction calculated. Margination of granulocytes was similar prior to (21.5% $\pm$ 13.4%) and during infusion (23.3% $\pm$ 9.6%) of rHuGM-CSF.

The ability of granulocytes to migrate to a peripheral sterile, inflammatory site was measured using a standardized skin chamber assay[11 12] in 15 patients before chemotherapy and autologous bone marrow transplantation (baseline). Ten of these patients were again studied during continuous infusion of rHuGM-CSF at a time when the peripheral leukocyte count was comparable to baseline; three patients treated with high dose chemotherapy and autologous bone marrow support but who did not receive rHuGM-CSF were also studied at the time of hematopoietic recovery as controls. Migration of granulocytes to a sterile inflammatory site use a standardized skin chamber assay [13 14] was markedly reduced during continuous rHuGM-CSF infusion (1.2 $\pm$ 0.9 WBC/cm^2/24 hours) compared to baseline (39.6 $\pm$ 17.7 WBC/cm^2/24 hours; $p < 0.0008$) [15].

Effect of rHuGM-CSF on Phagocytosis and Oxidative Burst

We next analyzed the ability of the granulocytes maturing during rHuGM-CSF infusion to phagocytize ^{35}S-labelled *Cryptococcus neoformans*. The serum dependent ingestion of *Cryptococcus neoformans* was enhanced during administration of rHuGM-CSF compared to patients prior to chemotherapy and rHuGM-CSF administration and similar in patients not receiving rHuGM-CSF but the same high dose chemotherapy and bone marrow support.

Granulocytes exert a major portion of their killing function through the generation of reactive oxygen reduction products. We measured the basal and phorbol myristate acetate (PMA) stimulated production of hydrogen peroxide in patients prior to and during administration of rHuGM-CSF. These experiments demonstrated that hydrogen peroxide production in response to PMA is similar in granulocytes obtained from patients without and during rHuGM-CSF treatment.

DISCUSSION

Recombinant granulocyte-macrophage colony stimulating factor has been demonstrated in these studies to accelerate hematopoietic recovery in patients receiving high dose combination alkylating agents and autologous bone marrow support. Further, compared to a historical control population, there were fewer bacteremias, and fewer treatment related complications in patients receiving rHuGM-CSF. While these results require confirmation in a prospective, randomized clinical trial, they provide incentive for continued study. However, the data also demonstrate that rHuGM-CSF administration to man has effects on multiple stages of myeloid maturation.

Of importance however, is the inability of even very high doses of GM-CSF to eliminate the absolute leukopenia seen early on in the transplant setting. There appears to be an absolute requirement for a given period of time for maturation of the "stem" cell to committed progenitors before the GM-CSF can be effective. This observation, coupled with the fact that the majority of infections occurred during this time frame, suggests that the major effect of GM-CSF is on a committed progenitor and that efforts to alter this response will require will require either the use of factors acting earlier in the differntiation schema, or provision of additional progenitors that are susceptible to GM-CSF action.

It is important to remember that the measurement of peripheral leukocytes by conventional means may well underestimate host defense capacity. A common clinical experience is that severely neutropenic patients begin to clinically improve often several days prior to the appearance of circulating leukocytes suggesting that the peripheral leukocyte count may not be a complete measure of host defense. In the end, only a randomized, comparative trial will establish the utility of these growth factors as clinical adjuncts in severely myelosuppressed patients.

The reduced granulocyte mobilization to a sterile inflammatory site seen during continuous rHuGM-CSF infusion is consistent with known biological properties of this agent. Granulocyte macrophage colony stimulating factor has been shown to possess concentration dependent chemotaxis properties[16]. Further, GM-CSF has been shown to be equivalent to neutrophil inhibition factor (NIF-T) which results in decreased granulocyte migration in agar. Hence, continuous intravenous infusion of rHuGM-CSF would be expected to attract granulocytes to the peripheral blood because of the concentration gradient, but limit the migration to tissues due to NIF-T like activity. The partial recovery of granulocyte migration after discontinuation of rHuGM-CSF is consistent with this interpretation. These data would suggest that continuous intravenous infusion may not be the optimal manner of administration. A detailed analysis of the effects of bolus and continuous infusion GM-CSF of granulocyte migration is in progress. Similar inhibition of neutrophil migration has not been seen with G-CSF[17 18].

The clinical data of reduced bacteremias during rHuGM-CSF infusion is consistent with the presence of activated granulocytes in the peripheral blood. Fortunately, soft tissue infections in these patients are rare and might be expected to be increased if rHuGM-CSF paralysis of granulocyte migration detected by this assay is relevant to this type of infection. Other mechanisms, however, may be operative. It may be that rHuGM-CSF has effects on cells other than marrow and circulating granulocytes, such as tissue macrophages, and that stimulation of these cells would lead to enhanced host defense. Further detailed investigation will be required.

Nonetheless, the data caution that the peripheral leukocyte count alone should not be considered a sole determinant of the capacity of host defense and that the administration of pharmacologic doses of recombinant growth factors may have unexpected effects on the functional capacity of effector cells.

Acknowledgements

We thank the nurses, fellows and housestaff of the Duke University Bone Marrow Transplant Unit for their assistance in carrying out these studies. Supported in part by a grant from the Sandoz Research Institute. This work is not supported by a NIH grant.

References

1 Brandt SJ, Peters WP, Atwater SK, Kurtzberg J, Borowitz MJ, Jones RB, Shpall EJ, Bast RC, Gilbert CJ and Oette DH. Effect of recombinant human granulocyte-macrophage colony-stimulating factor on hematopoietic reconstitution after high-dose chemotherapy and autologous bone marrow transplantation. New Engl J Med **318**: 869-876, 1988.

2 Peters WP, Shogan J, Shpall EJ, Jones RB, Kim CS: Recombinant human granulocyte-macrophage colony-stimulating factor produces fever. Lancet 1: 950, 1988

3 Shogan JE, Brandt SJ, Jones RB, Shpall EJ, Gilbert CJ, Atwater SK, Borowitz MJ, Bast RC, Kurtzberg J, Oette DH, and Peters WP. Toxicity from recombinant human granulocyte-macrophage colony stimulating factor (rHuGM-CSF) after high dose chemotherapy and autologous bone marrow transplant (ABMT). Proc Am Soc Can Research, 29: 53 (209) 1988.

4 Atwater, SJ, Borowitz M and Peters WP: Unpublished Observations.

5 Peters WP, Brandt SJ, Atwater SK, Borowitz MJ, Kurtzberg J, Jones RB, Shpall EJ, Shogan J, Bast RC, Oette DH. Effect of recombinant human granulocyte macrophage colony-stimulating factor (rHuGM-CSF) on hematopoietic reconstitution and granulocyte function following high dose chemotherapy (HDC) and autologous bone marrow transplantation (ABMT). Proc Am Soc Clin Oncol, 7:160 (C616) 1988.

6 Donahue RE, Wang EA, Stone DK, Kamen R, Wong GG, Sehgal PK, Nathan DG, and Clark SC: Stimulation of hematopoiesis in primates by continuous infusion of recombinant human GM-CSF. Nature 321:872-875, 1986.

7 Groopman JE, Mitsuyasu RT, DeLeo MJ, Oette DH, Golde DW. Effect of recombinant human granulocyte-macrophage colony-stimulating factor on myelopoiesis in the acquired immunodeficiency syndrome. N Engl J. Med 317: 593-598, 1987.

8 Vadhan-Raj S, Keating M, LeMaistre A, et al. Effects of recombinant human granulocyte-macrophase colony-stimulating factor in patients with myelodysplastic syndromes. N Engl J Med 317:1545-1552, 1987.

9 Nienhuis AW, Donahue RE, Darlsson S, Clark SC, Agricola B, Antinoff N, Pierce JE, Turner P, Anderson WF and Nathan DG. Recombinant human granulocyte-macrophage colony-stimulating factor (GM-CSF) shortens the period of neutropenia after autologous bone marrow transplantation in a primate mode. J Clin Invest **80**: 573, 1987.

10 Gasson JC, Weisbart RH, Kaufman SE, Clark SC, Hewick RM, Wong GG, Golde DW. Purified human granulocyte-macrophage colony-stimulating factor: Direct action of neutrophils. Science **226**: 1339-1342, 1984.

11 Senn H, Holland JF, Bannerjee T. Kinetic and comparative studies on localized leukocyte mobilization in normal man. J Lab Clin Med **74**: 742, 1969.

12 Peters WP, Holland JF, Senn HJ, Rhomberg W, Banerjee T. Corticosteroids and localized leukocyte mobilization. New Engl J Med **282**: 342, 1972.

13 Senn H, Holland JF, Bannerjee T. Kinetic and comparative studies on localized leukocyte mobilization in normal man. J Lab Clin Med **74**: 742, 1969.

14 Peters WP, Holland JF, Senn HJ, Rhomberg W, Banerjee T. Corticosteroids and localized leukocyte mobilization. New Engl J Med **282**: 342, 1972.

15 Peters WP, Stuart A, Affronti ML, Kim CS, Coleman RE. Neutrophil migration is defective during recombinant human granulocyte-macrophage colony stimulating factor (rHuGM-CSF) infusion after autologous bone marrow transplantation in man. Blood 72:1310-1315, 1988.

16 Wang JM, Collella S, Allavena P, Mantovani A. Immunology 60: 439-333, 1987.

17 Toner GC, Jakubowski AA, Crown JP, Peters WP, Souza L, Gabrilove JL: Neutrophil migration in pateints receiving rhG-CSF. Blood 72: 154a, 1988.

18 Peters WP, Kurtzberg J, Atwater S, Borowitz M, Gilbert C, Rao M, Currie M Shogan J, Jones RB, Shpall EJ, Stead R, Souza L: Comparative effects of rHuG-CSF and rHuGM-CSF on hematopoietic reconstitution and granulocyte function following high dose chemotherapy and autologous bone marrow transplantation (ABMT). Proc ASCO 8: 16, 1989.

Hematopoietic Growth Factors
in Transfusion Medicine, pages 129–141

CELLULAR INTERACTION REGULATING THE PRODUCTION OF COLONY-STIMULATING FACTORS

James D. Griffin, George D. Demetri, Yuzuru Kanakura, Stephen A. Cannistra, and Timothy J. Ernst

Division of Tumor Immunology, Dana-Farber Cancer Institute, Boston, MA 02115

INTRODUCTION

Blood cell formation is regulated by a complex network of cells and factors which maintain an enormous daily production of granulocytes, monocytes, erythrocytes, lymphocytes, and platelets. This system also provides a mechanism for the marrow to respond rapidly to a variety of emergencies ranging from blood loss to acute bacterial infection. Cells of all hematopoietic lineages are derived from a small pool of pluripotent, self-renewing, stem cells. Evidence for the existence of self-renewing stem cells first came from the work of Till and McCullouch, who noted almost 30 years ago that injection of syngeneic marrow into lethally irradiated mice resulted in the formation of macroscopic colonies of hematopoietic cells in the spleen (Till et al., 1961). The colonies were shown to be the product of single cells, termed **CFU-S** (colony forming unit-spleen), through the use of marker chromosomes. Moreover, it was shown that CFU-S had the ability to self-renew since colonies could be excised, homogenized, and reinjected into new irradiated recipients resulting in the growth of new CFU-S colonies. At about the same time, Pluznick, Sachs, Pike, Robinson, Metcalf, and others initiated efforts to define *in vitro* culture conditions which would support growth of hematopoietic precursor cells (Bradley et al., 1966; Ichikawa et al., 1966; Pike et al., 1970). In semi-solid media, marrow cells exhibited very little spontaneous proliferation, but colonies of single or multiple lineages were readily produced in when "colony-stimulating factors" were added (initially in the form of media conditioned by exposure to lectin-stimulated spleen cells, mononuclear blood cells, or certain tumor cell lines). The *in vitro* assays continue to be refined, but have made it possible to identify a hierarchy of hematopoietic progenitor cells and determine their individual growth factor requirements. The most primitive and most recently identified clonogenic cell has been termed the **CFU-Blast** by Ogawa and colleagues (Suda et al., 1983; Leary et al., 1987; Rowley et al., 1987), and is a cell which gives rise to a small colony composed of blasts with a high secondary plating efficiency. The CFU-Blast cell also has some degree of self-renewal. Evidence from murine marrow transplantation studies suggest that blast colony cells are very close to true hematopoietic (transplantable) stem cells. The recent efforts of Weissman and colleagues to purify murine hematopoietic stem cells are likely to clarify the relationship of CFU-S and CFU-Blast to true stem cells (Spangrude et al., 1988). Several other distinct stages of progenitor cells have been identified which fall between stem cells and mature myeloid elements. The **CFU-GEMM** is a cell which is multipotent by virtue of its ability to give rise to multiple cell lineages (granulocyte, erythrocyte, monocyte, megakaryocyte) but one which has a very limited capacity for self-renewal (Fauser et al., 1979). Careful morphologic analysis of CFU-GEMM colonies, particularly in the mouse, has demonstrated the existence of many "intermediate" forms in which virtually any combination of two or three lineages can be found, and some investigators interpret such results as evidence for "stochastic" differentiation (Leary et al., 1987; Suda et al., 1984; Suda et al., 1984; Leary et al., 1985; Ogawa et al., 1983). In general, however, the events regulating lineage commitment of progenitor cells both *in vitro* and *in vivo* are not well understood. Several different levels of progenitor cells committed to granulocyte/monocyte differentiation can be identified, and will produce colonies containing only neutrophils, both neutrophils and monocytes, only monocytes, or only eosinophils.

These cells, termed **CFU-G, CFU-GM, CFU-M, or CFU-Eo,** respectively, have not self-renewal potential and a high fraction are actively cycling (Cannistra et al., 1988). Similarly, clonogenic cells committed to erythroid differentiation can be assayed as burst forming units **(BFU-E)** or the more mature **CFU-E** (McLeod et al., 1974). While the development of *in vitro* and *in vivo* assays for hematopoietic progenitor cells have led to significant advances in our understanding of myelopoiesis, there remains a great deal to learn about the events which regulate both basal hematopoiesis and stress hematopoiesis.

The conditioned media which were originally used to support the growth of clonogenic cells have been shown to contain several specific factors. A number of factors have been shown to act directly on progenitor cells to stimulate production of neutrophils and/or monocytes, including interleukin 3 (IL-3), granulocyte macrophage CSF (GM-CSF), granulocyte CSF (G-CSF), and macrophage CSF (M-CSF, or CSF-1) (Metcalf et al., 1986; Sieff et al., 1987). A number of other factors, including IL-1, IL-4, IL-5, and IL-6, also are likely to have important direct and indirect effects on many aspects of myelopoiesis, including a direct proliferative activity on CFU-Blast and CFU-GEMM cells (IL-1, IL-6, and possibly G-CSF also), regulation of eosinophil production (IL-5), regulation of mast cell development (IL-4), and regulation of cytokine release by accessory cells (IL-1, IL-4, IL-6). The cDNAs for all of the CSF genes have been cloned and recombinant human and murine factors produced (Clark et al., 1987; Yang et al., 1986; Wong et al., 1985; Souza et al., 1986; Kawasaki et al., 1985; Wong et al., 1987; Nagata et al., 1986). The availability of pure CSFs has allowed very precise characterization of their functions and specificity. The cellular targets of IL-3, GM-CSF, G-CSGF, and M-CSF are summarized in Figure 1.

IL-3 and GM-CSF are broadly active factors which can stimulate proliferation of cells as early as the CFU-Blast. Both factors are good stimulators of BFU-E and CFU-GM. It seems likely that IL-3 is modestly more potent on earlier cells than GM-CSF, and that GM-CSF is modestly more potent than IL-3 on later cells. As single factors, M-CSF and G-CSF act primarily to promote development of monocytes or neutrophils. respectively. However, G-CSF may also have some activity, at least *in vitro*, on early progenitor cells, particularly in combination with other CSFs. *In vivo*, however, G-CSF administration appears to cause almost exclusively neutrophilia, without evidence of increased red cell or platelet production (Welte et al., 1987; Cohen et al., 1987; Gabrilove et al., 1988; Bronchud et al., 1987). This is also, however, true for GM-CSF, despite the clear ability of this

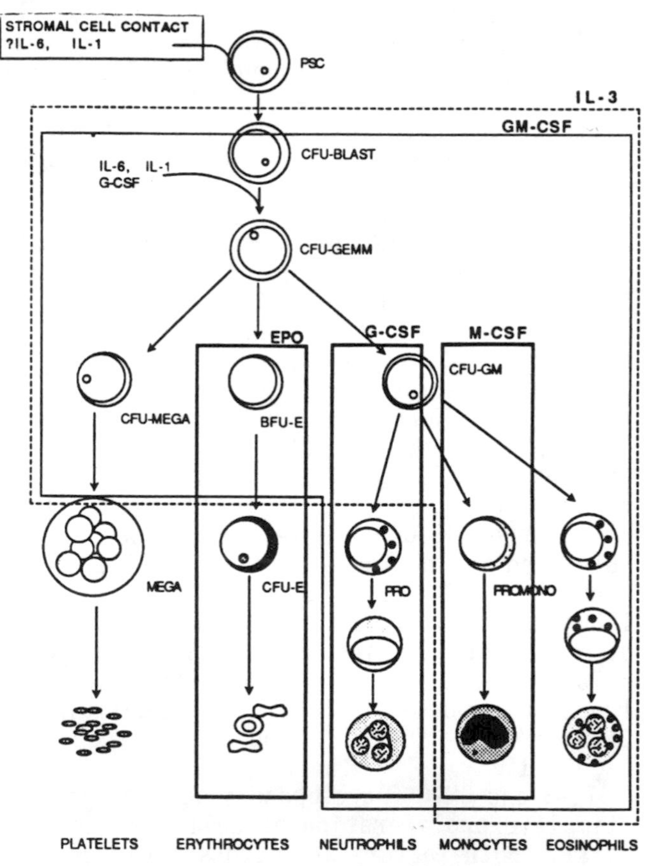

FIGURE 1. SUMMARY OF THE ACTIVITY OF CSFs ON HEMATOPOIESIS.

factor to promote proliferation of CFU-GEMM and BFU-E *in vitro*. Human trials with IL-3 have not been reported at this time, but animal studies suggest that the factor may have broader effects on hematopoiesis than GM-CSF (Metcalf et al., 1986; Donahue et al., 1988). Administration of M-CSf to non-human primates causes a monocytosis. Humans have been treated with M-CSf partially purified from urine, and increases in leukocyte count have been observed (Motoyoshi et al., 1986). In mice, M-CSF induces a substantial increase in the fraction of CFU-GM in the cell cycle (Broxmeyer et al., 1987; Broxmeyer et al., 1987). The ability of

SOURCES OF COLONY STIMULATING FACTORS

The known sources and inducers of specific CSFs are outlined in **Table 1**.

Table 1 Cellular Sources of CSFs

CELL LINEAGE	INDUCER*	CSF PRODUCED
T lymphocyte	TPA, PHA	GM-CSF, IL-3
T lymphocyte	anti-CD2	GM-CSF, IL-3
T lymphocyte	ionomycin	GM-CSF, IL-3
T lymphocyte	IL-1	GM-CSF
monocyte	TPA-CHX	G-CSF, M-CSF
monocyte	LPS	G-CSF
monocyte	GM-CSF, IL-3	M-CSF
fibroblasts	TNF, IL-1	GM-CSF, G-CSF
fibroblasts	PDGF	M-CSF
mesothelial	EGF, TNF, LPS	GM-CSF, G-CSF
endothelial	TNF, IL-1	GM-CSF, G-CSF, M-CSF
glial cells	none	IL-3
mast cells	IgE, A23187	IL-3, GM-CSF

* TPA = tetradeconoyl 13-phorbal ester; PHA = phytohemagglutinin; CHX = cycloheximide; LPS = lipopolysaccharide; PDGF = platelet-derived growth factor; EGF = epidermal growth factor

GM-CSF and G-CSF to accelerate recovery of hematopoiesis following cytotoxic chemotherapy is impressive (Gabrilove et al., 1988; Bronchud et al., 1987; Antman et al., 1988) and adds further weight to the potential natural role of these factors in the regulation of hematopoiesis in stress situations.

There are several notable points. First, although many cells can produce CSFs, different CSFs are produced by different cells. For example, the T lymphocyte appears to be the primary source of IL-3, although neural cells in the murine cerebellum have recently been shown to have IL-3 transcripts (Ihle et al., 1983; Farrar et al., 1989). Activated T cells can also produce GM-CSF, but not G-CSF or M-CSF (Herrmann et al., 1988). Second, there is little evidence for constitutive production of CSFs, with the possible exception that most fibroblast cell lines produce M-CSF spontaneously. In all other circumstances, the production od CSFs is highly regulated primarily by mediators of inflammation such as endotoxin, TNF, y-interferon, IL-1, and IL-6 (Broudy et al., 1986; Munker et al., 1986; Bagby et al., 1986; Koeffler et al., 1988; Chan et al., 1988; Thorens et al., 1987; Vellenga et al., 1988; Ernst et al., 1989). Thus, what is known about CSF gene regulation supports the notion that these growth factors are likely to play an important role in the hematopoietic response to infection or other stresses. Third, it is important to realize that the CSF genes can be independently regulated, even in the same cell type. For example, we have demonstrated that the blood monocyte can produce both G-CSF and M-CSF, and further that the stimuli inducing expression of each CSF are unique (Vellenga et al., 1988). Thus, exposure of monocytes to bacterial cell wall products (LPS) induces rapid expression of the G-CSF and secretion of G-CSF, while exposure of monocytes to T cell lympokines results in selective activation of the M-CSf gene. Both the M-CSF gene and the G-CSF gene can also be coordinately induced by factors such as cycloheximide and g-interferon. These results are summarized in Figure 2.

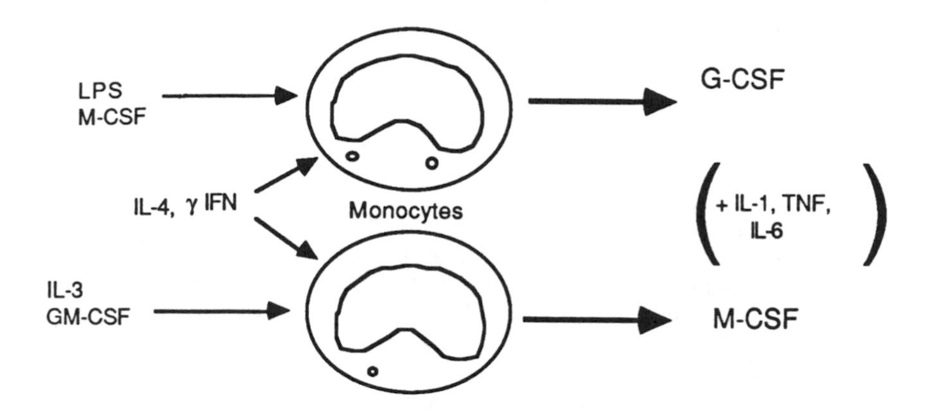

FIGURE 2. REGULATION OF CSF PRODUCTION BY NORMAL BLOOD MONOCYTES.

The mechanisms of CSF gene regulation are only partially understood, but have proven to be very interesting in several respects. In the majority of cell types investigated so far, transcription of the GM-CSF, G-CSF, and M-CSF genes is constitutive even in the absence of specific stimuli (Koeffler et al., 1988; Thorens et al., 1987; Ernst et al., 1989; Horiguchi et al., 1988). However, the transcripts which are produced are rapidly degraded in the cytoplasm and fail to accumulate or be translated into protein. The process of "induction" has been shown to be primarily due to stabilization of mRNAs, although small increases in transcriptional rates have also been observed. Also of interest is the fact that independent mechanisms have been demonstrated to stabilize transcripts of M-CSF and G-CSF in blood monocytes (Vellenga et al., 1988; Ernst et al., 1989). and also to independently stabilize transcripts for GM-CSF and *c-myc* in a murine monocytic tumor (Schuler et al., 1988). Even less is known about mechanisms to shut off CSF production. In human monocytes, G-CSF transcripts are automatically down-regulated approximately 18 hours after induction, by mechanisms which are yet to be determined (Ernst et al., 1989).

The activating signals for T cells involve mitogenic stimulae through the antigen receptor (either with specific antigen or by crosslinking of the T3 complex) or stimulation through the CD2 structure. There is evidence by *in situ* RNA hybridization that only a small fraction of blood T cells secrete GM-CSF or IL-3 (<5%) after stimulation. These results have recently been confirmed in our laboratory using *in situ* immunochemical demonstration of GM-CSF with monoclonal antibodies to this factor (Kanakura Y and Griffin JD, unpublished, 1989). There is evidence, however, that the IL-3 and GM-CSF genes may be independently regulated in T cells. The induction of GM-CSf gene transcription can be blocked by 1,25 $(OH)_2$ vitamin D3 (Tobler et al., 1987). The induction of IL-3 in T cells can be partially blocked by cyclosporine A (Bickel et al., 1987). The regulation of CSF production in T cells is summarized in Figure 3.

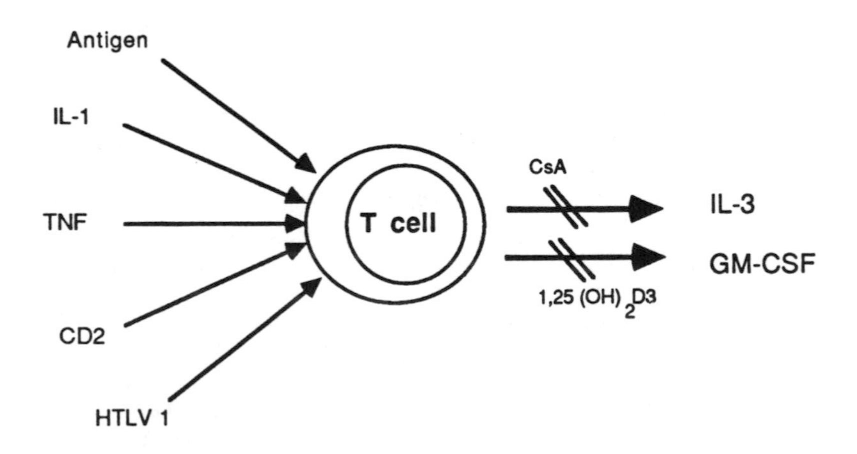

FIGURE 3. REGULATION OF CSF PRODUCTION BY NORMAL T LYMPHOCYTES.

Non-hematopoietic cells such as fibroblasts and endothelial cells are capable of secreting CSFs under many types of situations. Quiescent umbilical vein endothelial cells can be induced by IL-1, TNF, or LPS to secrete GM-CSF, G-CSF and M-CSF. Dermal fibroblasts spontaneously express M-CSF transcripts when cultured in serum-containing media. LPS and TNF induce expression of the G-CSF and GM-CSF genes. Epidermal growth factor (EGF) has little or no effect of CSF gene expression in these cells. In contrast, EGF has important effects on CSF gene expression in mesothelial cells (Demetri et al., 1989). EGF alone induces expression in cultured normal human peritoneal or pleural mesothelial cells, and acts synergistically with TNF to induce high level expression of both G-CSF and GM-CSF transcripts (Demetri et al., 1989).

There is a considerable degree of intercellular signaling resulting in a cascade of activation. Some of the possible interactions are summarized in Figure 4.

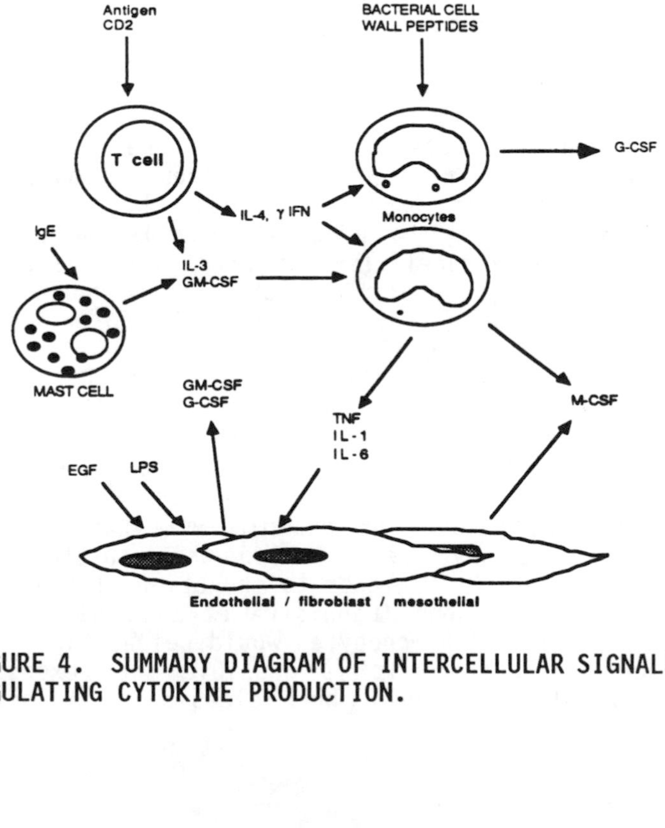

FIGURE 4. SUMMARY DIAGRAM OF INTERCELLULAR SIGNALLING REGULATING CYTOKINE PRODUCTION.

These results show that many cell types are capable of producing CSFs when stimulated with "inflammatory" cytokines or factors such as endotoxin. It is likely that this represents an important response system to infection or other acute events. It is further likely that local production of CSFs, by cells in the immediate area of inflammation, is important to attract and activate neutrophils, monocytes, eosinophils, and basophils. Some of the locally produced CSFs are likely to enter the vascular system and affect neutrophil margination, adhesiveness, release from the marrow, and, ultimately, increase production of granulocytes and monocytes by the marrow.

Many questions remain to be answered regarding the role of CSFs in the biology of hematopoiesis. The results presented above suggest an important role for CSFs in the response to infection or inflammation, but the role of CSFs in basal hematopoiesis remains to be determined. While marrow stromal cells can produce CSFs when stimulated, there is little evidence at present that there is any ongoing, constitutive, production of IL-3, GM-CSF, or G-CSF. It is possible that other factors or cell-cell interactions regulate basal hematopoiesis and that the CSFs are needed only to respond to stress. It is more likely, however, that basal blood cell production requires only very small amounts of CSFs, and that these will be delivered directly to progenitor cells by stromal cells or the extracellular matrix. *In situ* staining techniques with either RNA probes or immunochemical stains for the factors may prove informative in elucidating the role of CSFs in these situations.

With the increasing clinical use of the CSFs it is important that we gain a better understanding of the diverse effects of these factors on activation of mature myeloid cells and on non-hematopoietic cells. It is evident from Figure 4 that activation of a monocyte by GM-CSF, for example, may have complex effects. We have demonstrated that treatment of monocytes with GM-CSF leads to induction of the tumor necrosis factor gene (Cannistra et al., 1988). In situations in which monocytes would release TNF, such as acute infection, it is possible that excessive amounts of TNF could be released. A better understanding of the secondary effects of the CSFs may thus help to explain both some of the beneficial and toxic effects of the CSFs in patients.

ACKNOWLEDGEMENTS

This work was supported in part by PHS grants CA 36167 and CA 47843. J.D.G. is a Scholar of the Leukima Society of America.

REFERENCES

Antman KS, Griffin JD, Elias A, et al. N Engl J Med 319:593, 1988.
Bagby GC, Dinarello CA, Wallace P, et al. J Clin Invest 78:1316, 1986.
Bickel M, Tsuda H, Amstad P, Evequoz V, Mergenhagen SE, Wahl, Pluznik DH. Proc Natl Acad Sci 84:3274, 1987.
Bradley TR, Metcalf D. Aust J Exp Biol Med Sci 44:287, 1966.
Bronchud MH, Scarffe JH, Thatcher N, et al. Br J Cancer 56:809,1987.
Broudy VC, Kanshansky K, Segal GM, et al. Proc Natl Acad Sci USA 83:7467, 1986.
Broxmeyer HE, Williams DE, Cooper S, et al. J Clin Invest 79:721, 1987.
Broxmeyer HE, Williams DE, Hangoc G, et al. Proc Natl Acad Sci USA 84:3871, 1987.
Cannistra SA, Griffin JD. Semin Hematol 25:173, 1988.
Cannistra SA, Vellenga E, Rambaldi A, Griffin JD. Blood 71:672, 1988.
Chan JY, Slamon DJ, Nimer SD, et al. Proc Natl Acad Sci USA 83:8669, 1986.
Clark SC, Kamen R. Science 236:1229, 1987.
Cohen AM, Zsebo KM, Inoue H, et al. Proc Natl Acad Sci 84:2484, 1987.
Demetri GD, Zenzie BW, Rheinwald JG, Griffin JD. Blood, in press, 1989.
Donahue RE, Seehra J, Metzger M, et al. Science 241:1820, 1988.
Ernst TJ, Ritchie AR, Demetri GD, Griffin JD. J Biol Chem 264:5700, 1989.
Farrar WL, Vinocour M, Hell JM. Blood 73:137, 1989.

Fauser SS, Messner HA. Blood 53:1023, 1979.
Gabrilove JL, Jakubowski A, Scher H, et al. N Engl J Med 318:1414, 1988.
Herrmann F, Oster W, Meuer SC, et al. J Clin Invest 81:1415, 1988.

Horiguchi J, Sariban E, Kufe D. Mol Cell Biol 8:3951, 1988.
Ichikawa Y, Pluznick DH, Sachs L. Proc Natl Acad Sci 56:488, 1966.
Ihle JH, Keller J, Oroszlan S, et al. J Immunol 131:282, 1983.
Kawaski ES, Ladner MB, Wang AM et al. Science 230:291, 1985.
Koeffler HP, Gasson J, Tobler A. Mol Cell Biol 8:3432, 1988.
Leary AG, Ogawa M, Blood 69:953, 1987.
Leary AG, Strauss LC, Civin CI, Ogawa M. Blood 66:327, 1985.
McLeod DL, Shreve MM, Axelrad AA. Blood 44:517, 1974.
Metcalf D, Blood 67:257, 1986.
Metcalf D, Begley CG, Johnson GR, et al. Blood 68:46, 1986.
Motoyoshi K, Takaku F, Maekawa T, et al. Exp Hematol 14:1069, 1986.
Munker R, Gasson J, Ogawa M, Koeffler HP. Nature 323:79, 1986.
Nagata S, Tsuchiya M, Asano S, et al. J Exp Med 165:941, 1987.
Ogawa M, Porter PN, Nakahata T. Blood 61:823, 1983.
Pike BL, Robinson WA. J Cell Physiol 76:77, 1970.
Rowley SD, Sharkis SJ, Hattenburg C, Sensenbrenner LL. Blood 69:804, 1987.
Schuler GD, Cole MD. Cell 55:1115, 1988.
Sieff CA. J Clin Invest 79:1549, 1987.
Sprangrude GJ, Heinfeld S, Weissman IL. Science 241:58, 1988.
Suda J, Suda T, Ogawa M. Blood 64:393, 1984.
Suda T, Suda J, Ogawa M. Proc Natl Acad Sci USA 80:6689, 1986.
Suda T, Suda J, Ogawa M. Proc Natl Acad Sci USA 81:2520, 1984.
Thorens B, Mermound J, Vassalli P. Cell 48:671, 1987.
Till, JE, McCullough EA. Radiat Res 14:213, 1961.
Tobler A, Gasson J, Reichel H, Norman AW, Koeffler HP.

J Clin Invest 79:1700, 1987.
Vellenga E, Rambaldi A, Ernst T, et al. Blood 71:1528, 1988.
Wong GG, Witek JS, Temple PA, et al. Science 232:61. 1986.
Wong GG, Temple PA, Leary AC, et al. Science 235:1504, 1987.
Yang Y-C, Ciarletta AB, Temple PA et al. Cell 47:3, 1986.

Hematopoietic Growth Factors
in Transfusion Medicine, pages 143–150

Effects of Recombinant Human Granulocyte-Macrophage Colony-Stimulating Factor as Treatment for Aplastic Anemia and Agranulocytosis[1]

Richard E Champlin, Stephen D Nimer, Dagmar Oette, and David W Golde

UCLA Center for Health Sciences and the Jonsson Comprehensive Cancer Center Los Angeles, CA (R.E.C., S.D.N., D.W.G.) and Sandoz Research Institute, E. Hanover, NJ (D.O.)

INTRODUCTION

Aplastic anemia is a life-threatening hematologic disorder characterized by pancytopenia and a hypocellular bone marrow (Camitta et al, 1982). Patients with severe aplastic anemia have a poor prognosis without recovery of hematopoiesis.

A family of hematopoietic growth factors have been identified that stimulate proliferation of myeloid precursor cells _in vitro_. Granulocyte-macrophage colony-stimulating factor (GM-CSF) is a glycoprotein hormone that induces hematopoietic progenitors to form granulocyte, macrophage, and eosinophil colonies (Metcalf, 1986). Stimulatory activity for erythroid and megakaryocytic colony formation has been demonstrated under some circumstances. GM-CSF also has profound effects to enhance neutrophil function (Golde and Gasson, 1988). In vivo treatment with GM-CSF reduces leukocytosis in animals and enhances bone marrow recovery following cytotoxic chemotherapy treatment (Donahue et al, 1986).

Human GM-CSF has been molecularly cloned (Wong et al 1985) and parenteral treatment with GM-CSF has been studied

[1]Supported in part by PHS Grants CA-23175, CA 32737, CA-30388 and RR0685 from the United States Public Health Service

in a variety of disease states. Recombinant human granulocyte-macrophage colony-stimulating factor (rhGM-CSF) stimulates hematopoiesis *in vivo* in patients with AIDS (Groopman et al, 1987), myelodysplasia, (Vadhan-Raj et al, 1987), following myelotoxic chemotherapy (Antman et al, 1988) and following autologous bone marrow transplantation (Brandt et al, 1988). We evaluated rhGM-CSF as treatment for patients with refractory aplastic anemia (Champlin et al, 1989). This report summarizes our experience.

METHODS

Patients less than 75 years of age with acquired aplastic anemia who had previously failed to durably respond to antithymocyte globulin treatment were eligible if the bone marrow contained < 20% cellularity and 2 or more of the following were present: granulocytes < 1.0 x 10^9/l, reticulocytes < 60 x 10^9/l or platelets < 20 x 10^9/l. Patients with agranulocytosis with granulocytes < 1.0 x 10^9/l were also eligible. The study design was approved by the UCLA Human Subject Protection Committee. Informed consent was obtained from all patients or their legal guardians.

rhGM-CSF (Sandoz Corporation) with an activity of 5.4 x 10^6 units/mg glycoprotein was administered to groups of 3 or more patients by constant intravenous infusion through a central venous catheter for 14 days; if grade 2 or greater toxicity (Miller et al, 1981) did not occur, the dose was escalated to the next level for an additional 14 days. Patients with complete or partial responses continued on maintenance treatment at the same dose by constant intravenous infusion or subcutaneous injections for two additional months. Treatment was interrupted or discontinued for signs of toxicity. Patients with only a transient increment in granulocytes or less than a partial response after one month of therapy did not continue rhGM-CSF therapy. If 3 consecutive patients received a given dose level without toxicity, the succeeding group of patients was started at the next higher dose level. Dose levels ranged from 4 mcg/kg/d to 64 mcg/kg/d.

Complete response was defined as a sustained recovery of normal blood counts (granulocytes > 2.5 x 10^9/l, monocytes > 0.3 x 10^9/l, platelets > 150 x 10^9/l, Hb > 12 gm%). Partial response was defined as any of the following:

increment in granulocytes > 0.5 x 10^9/l above baseline; increment in monocytes > 0.2 x 10^9/l, increment in platelets > 30 x 10^9/l above baseline; or resolution of RBC transfusion requirements. Comparison was made for peripheral blood counts taken pretreatment and at day 28. The term granulocytes is operationally defined as the sum of segmented neutrophils plus band forms.

Progenitor assays for colony forming units-granulocyte, macrophage (CFU-GM) and burst forming units-erythropoiesis (BFU-E) on Ficoll/hypaque separated bone marrow and peripheral blood cells were performed in triplicates by standard techniques.

RESULTS

Fifteen patients were entered, 13 with aplastic anemia and 2 with agranulocytosis. Median age was 45 years (range 16-75 years). The etiology of aplastic anemia was unknown in 11, related to drugs in two and to hepatitis in one. Agranulocytosis was associated with the T-gamma syndrome in one patient and was idiopathic in the other case. The median interval from diagnosis to rhGM-CSF therapy was 333 (range 60-2120) days. Nine patients had previously failed to have any hematologic improvement following antithymocyte globulin treatment. For aplastic anemia patients, median (range) peripheral blood counts x 10^9/l were: leukocytes 1.7 (0.9-2.4); granulocytes 0.42 (0.03-0.77); lymphocytes 1.0 (0.46-2.2); monocytes 0.09 (0.02-.27); and platelets 5 (5-25). Median bone marrow cellularity was 3% with a range of 2-15%. Eleven patients with aplastic anemia received rhGM-CSF for more than one week and were evaluable for hematologic response. Two patients with aplastic anemia and both patients with agranulocytosis could not tolerate therapy and were evaluable for toxicity but not for hematologic response.

Ten of the eleven evaluable patients had a partial or complete response in granulocytes. Seven patients had complete responses and 3 had partial responses in granulocytes. After 28 days of rhGM-CSF therapy, the median increment for granulocytes was 1.8 x 10^9/l above baseline with a range of 0.2 to 9.0 x 10^9/l. The difference in pre- and post-treatment granulocytes was significant (p=0.01). The greatest increments occurred in patients with higher pre-treatment granulocyte counts, more cellular bone marrow and a greater number of pretreatment CFU-GM. For 7 patientswith initial granulocyte counts 0.30 to 0.77 x 10^9/l the median increment was 3.1 (range 1.4 - 9.0)x10^9/l. For 4 more severely granulocytopenic patients, the median increment was 0.9 (range 0.2 - 1.9). In one of these patients with severe aplasia the response was transient; granulocyte counts increased from 0.2 to 1.0 x 10^9/l, but returned to baseline after one month despite continuing rhGM-CSF. Granulocytosis was sustained in the remaining patients while rhGM-CSF was continued. The response was dose dependent; granulocyte counts decreased when the rhGM-CSF dose was reduced and fell to baseline levels after discontinuation of the drug. Monocytes increased from a baseline median (range) of .07 (.02-.15) x 10^9/l to .34 (.19-2.9)x 10^9/l (p=0.01). Five of the eight patients had monocyte increases into the normal range. Eosinophilia occurred in each patient. Eosinophil counts increased after approximately two weeks of therapy and typically equalled or exceeded granulocytes after four to six weeks of therapy. The median peak eosinophil count was 5.8 x 10^9/l with a range of 0.6 to 35.6x10^9/l. Lymphocyte counts fluctuated variably but no consistent changes were observed.

Erythrocytes, platelets and their transfusion requirements were unaffected except for one patient who had an increase in hemoglobin concentration from 7 to 11 gm/dl and in platelets from 20 to 45 x 10^9/l; these returned to baseline after rhGM-CSF was discontinued and responded to a second course of rhGM-CSF treatment.

Bone marrow cellularity increased in all evaluable patients with patchy areas of granulocytic and eosinophillic hyperplasia. Median (range) cellularity increased from 5% (2-15%) to 36% (10-55%) (p=0.01). No changes were apparent in erythroid precursors and megakaryocytes.

Committed myeloid progenitors, CFU-GM, were markedly reduced at study entry with a baseline median (range) of 8(1-28) per 2x10^5 bone marrow cells and 6(0-155)/ml in the peripheral blood. After 28 days of rhGM-CSF treatment, CFU-GM increased to 13 (1-41) per 2 x 10^5 bone marrow cells and 21(12-639)/ml in peripheral blood. The differences between pre- and post-treatment values is significant p=0.02. Peripheral blood BFU-E increased from a pretreatment value of 25(4-109)/ml to 40(17-400)/ml (p=0.02).

TOXICITY

No major toxicity occurred in three patients receiving 4 mcg/kg/d of rhGM-CSF followed by 8 mcg/kg/d. All patients complained of mild fatigue and myalgia, which were more prominent in patients receiving higher doses. Six patients received 16 mcg/kg/d. This dose was generally well tolerated but adverse effects did occur in patients who developed marked leukocytosis; two patients developed dyspnea and pulmonary infiltrates after 10 days and 5 weeks of rhGM-CSF therapy respectively.

Doses $\geq$ 32 mcg/kg were poorly tolerated. Patients frequently developed symptoms in areas of prior inflammation, such as recurrent jaundice in a patient with a past history of non-A, non-B hepatitis, and pericarditis in a man with a prior history of pericarditis 3 years earlier. A patient who had a colostomy because of a previous intraabdominal infection developed fever and abdominal pain when treated with rhGM-CSF at 32 mcg/kg/d. One patient tolerated 32 mcg/kg/d well for two weeks but developed pleuritis and pulmonary infiltrates after 5 days while receiving 64 mcg/kg/d. All adverse effects resolved quickly following discontinuation of rhGM-CSF.

Three patients developed hemorrhage which required discontinuation of rhGM-CSF therapy. These patients had severe thrombocytopenia which was refractory to platelet transfusions. These bleeding complications were probably unrelated to rhGM-CSF treatment.

DISCUSSION

This was study was designed to assess the toxicity and biologic effects in of rhGM-CSF in selected patients with refractory aplastic anemia. Results are similar to other recent studies (Antin et al, 1988; Nissen et al, 1988; Vadhan-Raj et al, 1988). Patients with the most severe aplasia had the least impressive response. Patients with > 0.3 granulocytes/microliter generally had substantial increases in the blood within 1-3 days and a progressive increase in granulocytic cells within the first 2-6 weeks of treatment. The bone marrow became increasingly cellular with granulocytic and eosinophillic hyperplasia. The prompt initial increase in circulating granulocytes probably resulted from mobilization and redistribution of cells or increased cell survival. The later increase was associated with increased proliferation of myeloid precursors reflected by bone marrow hyperplasia. Granulocyte, monocyte and eosinophil counts fell to baseline once rhGM-CSF was discontinued.

Only one patient had improvement in erythropoiesis and a modest increase in platelets. These findings conincide with the results of most animal and human studies in other settings where platelets were generally not effected.

The toxicity of rhGM-CSF was relatively mild and tolerable in doses up to 8 to 16 mcg/kg/d unless extreme leukocytosis occurred. Three patients with marked leukocytosis became symptomatic with severe myalgia or pulmonary infiltrates, possibly related either to a direct effect of GM-CSF or to the elevated levels of activated granulocytes and eosinophilis. At higher doses, myalgia, serositis, hepatitis and abdominal pain occurred in the absence of major changes in leukocyte counts. Patients often had manifestations of inflammation in previously diseased tissues. These adverse effects resolved promptly with discontinuation of rhGM-CSF.

These data indicate that rhGM-CSF induces granulocytosis and monocytosis in patients with refractory aplastic anemia. Continued treatment appears necessary to maintain the hematologic response. Further study is necessary to determine if longterm maintenance is necessary and if chronic treatment with rhGM-CSF will be effective and tolerable. Impaired migration of granulocytes has been reported in patients receiving GM-CSF (Peters et al, 1988). It is uncertain whether rhGM-CSF treatment will reduce the risk of infection. Controlled trials are necessary to determine whether rhGM-CSF will reduce morbidity and improve survival.

Growth factor therapies may ultimately be an effective treatment for aplastic anemia. The hematologic responses observed in this study indicate that in most patients, myeloid progenitors are present that are capable of proliferating in response to stimulatory agents. Since rhGM-CSF does not appear to have substantial effects on erythrocytes and megakaryocytes, therapy of aplastic anemia will likely require concomitant treatment with other hematopoietic growth factors which affect these cell lineages. During normal physiology, multiple growth factors influence hematopoiesis at various stages of differentiation. Treatment with multilineage stimulatory factors such as interleukin-3 alone or in combination with GM-CSF, interleukin-1, interleukin-6, erythropoietin and/or thrombopoietic factors may potentially prove more effective.

REFERENCES

Antin JH, Smith BR, Holmes W, Rosenthal DS (1988). Phase I/II study of recombinant human granulocyte-macrophage colony-stimulating factor in aplastic anemia and myelodysplastic syndromes. Blood 72:705-713.

Antman KS, Griffin JD, Elias A, et al (1988). Effect of recombinant human granulocyte-macrophage colony-stimulating factor on chemotherapy-induced myelosuppression. N Engl J Med 319:593-598.

Brandt SJ, Peters WP, Antwater SK, et al (1988). Effect of recombinant human granulocyte, macrophage-colony stimulating factor on hematopoietic reconstitution after high dose chemotherapy and autologous bone marrow transplantation. N Engl J Med 318:869-876.

Camitta BM, Storb R, Thomas ED (1982). Aplastic anemia: pathogenesis, diagnosis, treatment, and prognosis. N Engl J Med 306:645-52, 712-8.

Champlin R, Nimer SD, Oreland P, Oette DH, Golde DW (1989). Treatment of refractory aplastic anemia with recombinant human granulocyte-macrophage colony-stimulating factor. Blood 73:694-699.

Donahue RE, Wang EA, Stone, et al (1986). Stimulation of hematopoiesis in primates by continuous infusion recombinant human GM-CSF. Nature 321:872-875.

Golde DW, Gasson JC (1988). Cytokines: Myeloid growth factors. In Gallin JI, Goldstein IM, Snyderman R eds): "Inflammation: Basic Principles and Clinical Correlates," New York: Raven Press Ltd.

Groopman JE, Mitsuyasu RT, DeLeo MJ, Oette D, Golde DW (1987). Effect of recombinant human granulocyte-macrophage colony-stimulating factor on myelopoiesis in the acquired immunodeficiency syndrome. N Engl J Med 317:593-8.

Metcalf D (1986). The molecular biology and functions of the granulocyte-macrophage colony-stimulating factors. Blood 67:257-67.

Miller et al (1981). Criteria for toxicity and response. Cancer 47:207-14.

Nissen C, Tichelli A, Gratwohl, et al (1988). Failure of recombinant human granulocyte-macrophage colony-stimulating factor therapy in aplastic anemia patients with very severe neutropenia. Blood 72:2045-2047.

Peters WP, Stuart A, Affronti ML, et al (1988). Neutrophil migration is defective during recombinant human granulocyte-macrophage colony-stimulating factor infusion after autologous bone marrow transplantation in humans. Blood 72:1310-1315.

Vadhan-Raj S, Keating M, LeMaistre A, et al (1987). Effects of recombinant human granulocyte-macrophage colony-stimulating factor in patients with myelodysplastic syndromes. N Engl J Med 317:1545-52.

Vadhan-Raj S, Buescher S, LeMaistre A, et al (1988). Stimulation of hematopoiesis in patients with bone marrow failure and in patients with malignancy by recombinant human granulocyte macrophage colony-stimulating factor. Blood 72:134-141.

Wong GG, Witek JS, Temple PA, et al (1985). Human GM-CSF: molecular cloning of the complementary DNA and purification of the natural and recombinant proteins. Science 228:810-15.

Hematopoietic Growth Factors
in Transfusion Medicine, pages 151–161

EFFECTS OF TREATMENT OF MYELODYSPLASTIC SYNDROMES WITH RECOMBINANT HUMAN GRANULOCYTE COLONY STIMULATING FACTOR

Peter Greenberg, Robert Negrin, Arnon Nagler, Larry Souza and Timothy Donlon

Stanford Medical Center, Stanford, CA and AMGen, Thousand Oaks, CA

INTRODUCTION

In vitro marrow hemopoietic cultures were utilized to determine the possible efficacy of recombinant human G-CSF for treating the refractory cytopenias present in the myelodysplastic syndromes (MDS). Our studies showed responsiveness of enriched hemopoietic precursors in vitro to the proliferative and granulocytic differentiative stimuli of G-CSF, generally without increased clonal self-generation. In our Phase I/II trial, 17 patients have been treated for 2 months with subcutaneous administration (0.1 - 3ug/kg/day) of G-CSF, escalating doses every 2 weeks. This study indicated normalization of neutrophil counts in 15 patients and reticulocyte responses with decreased RBC transfusion requirements in 3 of 12 transfusion dependent patients. Marrow myeloid maturation improved in the responding patients. Extended treatment for additional 6-12 month periods has indicated persisting responses. This therapy was well tolerated without serious toxicity being noted. In vitro neutrophil function (chemotaxis and phagocytosis) remained normal or improved in 6 of 8

This work was supported in part by USPHS grant CA36915 from the National Institutes of Health, Veterans Administration Research Funds and AMGen tested patients. Transformation to AML has occurred in 1 RAEB-T patient during or within a month of the treatment period. Marrow cytogenetic studies indicate persistence of the initial normal and/or abnormal clones. These data demonstrate hematologic improvement in a substantial proportion of MDS patients and support the need for Phase III controlled trials to determine whether the natural history of these disorders is altered by administration of G-CSF.

The myelodysplastic syndromes (MDS) provide a clinical setting for evaluating the evolution of a relatively benign hematologic disorder into one that is frankly malignant. Patients with this disease have refractory cytopenias with associated cellular dysfunction whose marrows show morphologically defective myeloid maturation with dysplasia in at least two of the three hemopoietic cell lines. The course of these patients is relatively indolent. Infection and hemorrhage are the major causes of death and are associated with the patients' dominant cytopenias. However, in 10-40% of patients acute blastic transformation occurs (Jacobs et al., 1986; Greenberg et al., 1983). In assessing biologic features of these disorders clonal abnormalities have been demonstrated by in vitro marrow culture, marrow cytogenetic studies and molecular analysis of the hemopoietic cells (Greenberg et al., 1986; LeBeau et al., 1986; Janssen et al., 1989).

MDS patients have been categorized morphologically by the French, American and British (FAB) Cooperative Group as refractory anemia (RA), with ringed sideroblasts (RARS), refractory anemia with excess blasts (RAEB), RAEB in transformation (RAEB-T) and chronic myelomonocytic leukemia (CMML). RA and RARS patients, who have a lower degree of marrow myeloid maturation abnormalities than patients with RAEB or RAEB-T, generally have better prognosis than these latter individuals (Jacobs et al., 1986; Greenberg et al., 1983; Bennett et al., 1982; Mufti et al., 1985; Foucar et al., 1987; Kerhofs et al., 1987). Biologic markers such as in vitro marrow cell clonogenic assays and cytogenetics, have also been useful in assessing certain critical pathogenetic features in these disorders (Greenberg et al., 1986). Uncoupling between proliferative and differentiative programs in hemopoietic stem cells has been proposed as a basic biologic lesion in patients with MDS and leukemia (Lotem et al., 1982). Because of this cellular defect, maturation-inducing agents such as retinoic acid, vitamin D and low doses of cytosine arabinoside have been used in preclinical and clinical trials to treat MDS and myeloid leukemia. Studies in animal models with these agents have indicated that leukemic cell growth is diminished concomitant with enhanced defferentiation of these abnormal cells (Sachs et al., 1978; Lotem et al., 1981; Metcalf et al., 1982). Although effective in a small proportion of patients, these maturation-inducing agents have had little impact on effectively managing MDS (Koeffler et al., 1988; Chesson et al., 1986). Other therapeutic options have been suboptimal and current approaches are limited to supportive care such as red cell transfusions and antibiotics.

The development of in vitro marrow clonogenic culture assays led to discovery of a family of interacting hematopoietic growth factors - the colony stimulating factors (CSFs) -which have recently been demonstrated to have critical physiologic roles for controlling hemopoiesis in vivo (Metcalf et al., 1986). Multi-CSF (interleukin 3) and GM-CSF (granulocyte-monocyte CSF) have predominantly proliferative effects on early hemopoietic cell compartments whereas G-CSF and M-CSF have major differentiative as well as proliferative effects on later more lineage-restricted precursor cells (for granulocytes and monocytes, respectively). Each hemopoietic cell lineage appears to be regulated by both proliferative and differentiative stimuli. These functional human CSFs are now available in recombinant form. Marrow culture studies in MDS have demonstrated subnormal clonal growth and defective cellular maturation of myeloid and erythroid precursors which become more abnormal as these patients evolve towards AML (Greenberg et al., 1983). The presence of abnormal marrow cytogenetics or defective in vitro myeloid clonogenicity has been shown to have negative prognostic import in MDS (Greenberg et al., 1986; LeBeau et al., 1986).

Defective proliferation of hemopoietic precursors within MDS marrow has been suggested as being due to either decreased responsiveness to or decreased production of such hemopoietic factors. However, as some leukemic cells have enhanced proliferative responses of the CSFs in vitro (Metcalf et al., 1986; Miyauchi et al., 1987; Vellenga et al., 1987) concern exists regarding the safety of using such agents in responsive neoplastic cells. Therefore, in order to evaluate the proliferative vs. differentiative responsiveness of hemopoietic precursors in MDS to hemopoietic growth factors and determine the possible clinical utility of CSF treatment we assessed in vitro proliferative, differentiative and self-generative responses of marrow cells from these patients to G-CSF and GM-CSF.

RESULTS

The proliferative and differentiative effects of recombinant human G-CSF and GM-CSF on marrow hemopoietic precursors from 17 MDS patients and 9 normal subjects were evaluated using methylcellulose clonogenic and liquid suspension culture assays (Nagler et al., 1987; Nagler et al., 1985). Enriched immature myeloid cell populations (EIMCP) (consisting of approximately 90% myeloblasts and promyelocytes and 10% lymphocytes, containing the hemopoietic progenitor cells) were obtained by removing nonadherent buoyant bone marrow cells by "panning" with anti-My8 and anti-glycophorin antibodies (Greenberg et al., 1985). These nonbound EIMCP were plated in clonogenic culture to assess hemopoietic colony formation (CFU-GM, BFU-E). After 7 day liquid culture with 5nM recombinant human G-CSF or GM-CSF (AMGen), placental conditioned medium or saline alone myeloid differentiation was assessed morphologically and secondary plating for clonogenicity (to assess hemopoietic progenitor cell self-generation) was performed (Nagler et al., 1987; Nagler et al., 1985; Nagler et al., 1988; Nagler et al., 1989).

CFU-GM and BFU-E were subnormal in 13 of 17 patients. After liquid culture with either G-CSF or GM-CSF decreased myeloid clonal self generation was noted in 11 of 13 patients, associated with enhanced myeloid differentiation. For normal marrow cells rhG-

CSF induced greater granulocytic differentiation than did rhGM-CSF (32% vs. 18% of the cells ,$p < 0.05$). Neutrophilic induction (> 10% mature neutrophils) occurred in 87% vs. 69% of control subjects with G-CSF and GM-CSF respectively. For the MDS patients G-CSF also induced greater granulocytic differentiation than did GM-CSF (8% vs. 1%, $p < 0.05$). Neutrophilic induction occurred in 46% vs. 24% of MDS patients respectively. GM-CSF showed enhanced monocytic differentiation potential compared to rhG-CSF both for normals and MDS patients. However, as monocytic differentiation occurred in the liquid cultures with medium alone the monocytic differentiative effect of G-CSF both in normals and MDS patients appears to be minimal. The granulocytic differentiation effect of G-CSF was less potent for the MDS patients than for normals (8 vs. 32%, respectively, $p < 0.05$) Dose response curves of MDS marrow cells with G-CSF and GM-CSF for these colony forming cells demonstrated normal to increased proliferative sensitivity in MDS cases to GM-CSF vs. normal to decreased proliferative responses to G-CSF. Four patients demonstrated characteristic cytogenetic abnormalities. After 7 days of liquid culture in the presence of G-CSF their EIMCP in vitro expressed the same karyotypic abnormalities as the native BM cells, suggesting induced differentiation by these factors of the abnormal clones (Nagler et al., 1987; Nagler et al., 1985; Nagler et al., 1988; Nagler et al, 1989).

These data utilizing in vitro culture techniques provided a biologic framework defining MDS marrow cell myeloid differentiative responsiveness to G-CSF without excessive clonal self-generation. These findings suggested possible efficacy and safety of G-CSF in this setting and led to our Phase I/II therapeutic protocol treating MDS patients with recombinant human G-CSF from AMGen. The design of the protocol was to evaluate clinical and biologic parameters, peripheral blood counts, in vitro neutrophil function, bone marrow morphology, cytogenetics and in vitro myeloid cell growth, assessing responsiveness to the CSFs. We treated 17 MDS patients (2 refractory anemia, 9 RAEB, 6 RAEB-T) with daily subcutaneous (SQ) injections of G-CSF, escalating dosage levels every two weeks from 0.1-3.0 ug/kg/day for a 6-8 week period (Negrin et al., 1989;

Negrin et al., 1989; Negrin et al., 1989). Fifteen patients have had significant elevations in both WBC (1.6-10 fold) and absolute neutrophil counts (ANC, 5-40 fold). Nine of 11 severely neutropenic patients (ANC < 500/mm^3) had rises in ANC to 1200-16,300 cells/mm^3. All 7 moderately neutropenic patients (ANC 500-1800/mm^3) had rises in ANC 5-16 fold. In 5 patients a greater than two-fold rise in reticulocyte counts occurred and 3 of 12 RBC transfusion-dependent patients had a decrease in RBC requirements. Improved marrow myeloid maturation was noted in 15 of 17 patients. In vitro neutrophil function (phagocytosis and chemotaxis) either remained normal or improved after treatment in 6 of 8 patients. Native marrow cytogenetic abnormalities, initially present in 4 responding patients, persisted after treatment, suggesting that enhanced differentiation of the abnormal clone occurred. These findings parallelled the in vitro results. No significant changes in platelet, lymphocyte, monocyte or eosinophil counts were found during treatment in 16 of 17 patients. After discontinuing G-CSF treatment following the initial 2 month treatment period peripheral WBCs returned to baseline levels over 2-4 weeks (Negrin et al., 1989; Negrin et al., 1989; Negrin et al., 1989). Toxicity was minimal, with only 2 patents stopping G-CSF injections because of side effects related to pre-existing clinical conditions (psoriasis, nausea and anorexia). One patient initially had RAEB-T converted to acute myeloid leukemia (AML) during this initial study. In this individual pre-treatment in vitro in culture had revealed a marked increase in proliferative sensitivity of his hemopoietic precursors to G-CSF and GM-CSF associated with increased CFU-GM self generation and poor myeloid differentiation in vitro. Transient increases in blast counts occurred in two patients and mild fluid overload in one patient. In several patients other medical problems occurred, likely related to their pre-existing cardiac or pulmonary disorders.

After the 2 month trial with G-CSF treatment we compared marrow proliferative and differentiative responses in vitro pre-and post-therapy using methylcellulose clonogenic and liquid suspension culture assays for hemopoietic precursors. Nine MDS patients, 8 of whom had marked neutrophil elevations with treatment were evaluated. Dose response curves for G-CSF and GM-CSF in vitro were similar in those obtained from patients prior to and after treatment with G-CSF. In one patient an increased proliferative sensitivity of these cells to both G-CSF and GM-CSF in vitro was noted. This patient was the individual who developed AML after treatment with G-CSF. Post treatment CFU-GM stimulated by G-CSF in vitro were increased in 7 of 9 evaluated patients and BFU-E (stimulated by Mo conditioned medium and erythropoietin) were increased in 4 of 5 patients compared to pretreatment values. G-CSF increased mature granulocyte differentiation in suspension culture in most patients post-as well as pre-treatment. Concomitant with enhanced in vitro differentiation of these MDS cells upon treatment with G-CSF, suppression of myeloid clonal self generation in vitro persisted (i.e 19% of basal levels post treatment after in vitro liquid culture exposure to G-CSF vs. 18% pre-treatment) (Nagler et al., 1988; Nagler et al., 1989).

As a result of the clinical responsiveness and tolerance of these patients to G-CSF the initial 2 month Phase I and II trial was extended, utilizing the same dose (generally 1 to 3 ug/kg/day) to which the patients initially responded. To date 9 patients have received this more extended therapy and 8 of the 9 patients have had improvements of their neutrophil counts which have persisted for at least 6 to 12 months (Negrin et al., 1989; Negrin et al., 1989). Two of four RBC transfusion-dependent patients had decreases in their transfusion requirements. Platelet counts were generally not altered by this therapy. Neutrophil function (in vitro chemotaxis and phagocytosis), which was maintained or improved after two months of treatment, was further augmented in 5 patients after an additional six months of G-CSF therapy.

These data indicated that G-CSF injected subcutanieously on a chronic basis was well tolerated and effective for persistent improvement in neutrophil counts and in vitro function, marrow myeloid maturation and possibly decreasing RBC transfusion requirements in MDS patients. One patient has developed AML and had strikingly abnormal in vitro proliferative and differentiative responses to G-CSF (see above) suggesting the possible prognostic import of such culture studies.

Cytogenetic abnormalities were found in 4 patients initially (one of whom had an enhanced differentiative response in vitro) and the remaining patients had normal cytogenetics. These findings generally persisted during G-CSF treatment. Eleven of 13 patients with normal marrow cytogenetics and the 4 patients with abnormal cytogenetics had improved neutrophil responses after therapy. The persisting cytogenetic abnormalities after treatment suggest that enhanced differentiation of the abnormal clone occurred.

In conclusion, these in vitro marrow clonogenic and suspension culture studies suggested the potential therapeutic utility of G-CSF for MDS patients. This analysis, based on the in vitro responsiveness to proliferative an myeloid differentiative stimuli without increased self-generation of the hemopoietic precursors, was subsequently shown to correlate with the high proportion of these patients whose marrow granulopoiesis and neutrophil levels responded to treatment. The in vivo and in vitro differentiative responses of marrow precursors from these patients suggest that decreased effective levels of G-CSF underlie certain cytopenias in MDS. These data indicate that Phase III controlled trials in MDS are warranted to assess the effects of G-CSF on survival, infectious episodes and evolution to AML.

REFERENCES

Bennett, JM, Catovsky D, Daniel MT, Flandrin G, Galton DAG, Gralnick HR & Sultan C. (FAB Cooperative Group) (1982). Proposals for the classification of the myelodysplastic syndromes. British Journal of Haematology 51:189.

Chesson BD, Jasperse DM, Simon R, et al (1986). A critical appraisal of low-dose cytosine arabinoside in patients with acute non-lymphocytic leukemia and myelodysplastic syndromes. J Clin Oncol 4:1857.

Foucar K, Langdon RM, Armitage JO, Olson DB & Carroll TJ (1985). Myelodysplastic syndromes. A clinical and pathologic analysis of 109 cases. Cancer 56:553.

Greenberg PL (1863). The smoldering myeloid leukemic states: Clinical and biologic features Review. Blood 61:1035.

Greenberg PL (1986). In vitro culture techniques defining biologic abnormalities in the myelodysplastic syndromes and myeloproliferative disorders. Clinics in Haematology 15:973.

Greenberg PL, Baker S, Link M, Minowada J (1985). Immunologic selection of hemopoietic precusor cells utilizing antibody-mediated plate binding ("panning"). Blood 65:190.

Jacobs RH, Cornbleet MA, Vardiman JW, et al (1986). Prognostic implications of morphology and karyotype in primary myelodysplastic syndromes. Blood 67:1765.

Janssen JWG, Buschle M, Layton M, Drexler NG, Lyons J, Van den Berghe H, Heimpel H, Kubanek B, Kleihauer E, Mufti GJ, Bartram CR (1989). Clonal analysis of myelodysplastic syndromes: evidence of multipotent stem cell origin. Blood 73:248.

Kerhofs H, Hermans J, Haak HL, and Leeksma CHW (1987). Utility of the FAB classification for myelodysplastic syndromes: investigation of prognostic factors in 237 cases. British Journal of Haematology 65:73.

Koeffler HP, Heitgan D, Mertelsmann R et al (1988). Randomized study of 13 cis-retinoic acid vs. placebo in the myelodysplastic disorders. Blood 71:703.

LeBeau MM, Albain KS, Larson R, et al (1986). Clinical and cytogenetic correlations in 63 patients with therapy-related myelodysplastic syndromes and acute nonlymphocytic leukemia: further evidence for characteristic abnormalities of chromosomes No. 5 and 7. J Clin Oncol 4:325.

Lotem J, Sachs L (1982). Mechanisms that uncouple growth and differentiation in myeloid leukemia cells: restoration of requirement for normal growth-inducing protein without restoring induction of differentiation-inducing protein. Proc Nat Acad Sci (USA) 79:4347.

Lotem J, Sachs L (1981). In vitro inhibition of the development of myeloid leukemia by injection of macrophage and granulocyte-inducing protein. Int J Cancer 28-375.
Metcalf D (1982). Regulator-induced suppression of myelomonocytic leukemic cells: Clonal analysis of early cellular events. Int J Cancer 38:121.
Metcalf D (1986). The molecular biology and functions of the granulocyte-macrophage colony-stimulating factors. Blood 67:257.
Miyauchi J, Kelleher CA, Yang YC, Wong GG, Clark SC, Minden MD, Minkin S, McCulloch EA (1987). The effects of three recombinant growth factors, IL-3, GM-CSF and G-CSF, on the blast cells of acute myeloblastic leukemia maintained in short term suspension culture. Blood 76:657.
Mufti GJ, Stevens JR, Oscier DG, Hamblin TJ & Machin D (1985). Myelodysplastic syndromes: a scoring system with prognostic significance. British Journal of Maematology 59:425.
Nagler A, Ginzton N, Bangs C, et al (1987). In vitro effects of recombinant human granulocyte and granulocyte-monocyte colony stimulating factors on hemopoiesis in the myelodysplastic syndromes. Blood 70 (suppl 1):140a.
Nagler A, Ginzton N, Bangs C Donlon T, Greenberg PL. In vitro differentiative and proliferative effects of human recombinant colony stimulating factors on marrow hemopoiesis in myelodysplastic syndromes. Leukemia (1990) in press.
Nagler A, Ginzton N, Negrin RS, Donlon T, Souza L, Greenberg PL (1988). In vitro hemopoiesis in myelodysplastic syndrome patients treated with recombinant human granulocyte colony stimulating factor. Blood 72 (suppl 1):128a.
Nagler A, Mackichan ML, Ginzton N, Negrin R, Donlon T, Bangs D, Greenberg PL (1989). In vitro responsiveness of marrow hemopoietic precursors in myelodysplastic syndromes following treatment with recombinant human G-CSF. Submitted.
Negrin RS, Haeuber DH, Nagler A, Donlon T, Greenberg P (1989). Treatment of myelodysplastic syndromes with recombinant human granulocyte colony stimulating factor. Ann Int Med 110:976.

Negrin RS, Haeuber DH, Nagler A, Donlon T, Souza L, Greenberg P (1989). Maintenance treatment of myelodysplastic syndromes with recombinant human granulocyte colony stimulating factor. Exp Hematol 17 (6):657a.

Negrin RS, Haeuber DH, Nagler A, Donlon T, Souza L, Greenberg P (1989). Effects of maintenance treatment of myelodysplastic syndromes with recombinant human granulocyte colony stimulating factor. Blood 74(Suppl 1):119a.

Sachs L (1978). Annotation: The differentiation of myeloid leukemia cells-new possibilities for therapy. Br J Haematol 40:509.

Vellenga E, Young DC, Wagner K, Wier D, Ostapovicz D, Griffin JD (1987). The effects of GM-CSF and G-CSF in promoting growth of clonogenic cells in acute myeloblastic leukemia. Blood 69:1771.

Hematopoietic Growth Factors
in Transfusion Medicine, pages 163–176

GRANULOCYTE MACROPHAGE COLONY STIMULATING FACTOR (GM-CSF) IN AIDS

DAVID T. SCADDEN, M.D.
NEW ENGLAND DEACONESS HOSPITAL
185 PILGRIM ROAD
BOSTON, MA 02215

The hematologic consequences of HIV infection are multiple including low peripheral blood cell counts, hypergammaglobulinemia and coagulation abnormalities. Cytopenias frequently limit anti-retroviral therapy as well as treatment for HIV-associated neoplasms and opportunistic infections. The use of agents which are capable of ameliorating low blood counts may therefore play an important adjunctive role in the care of AIDS patients.

BACKGROUND:

The causes of cytopenias in HIV infected patients may be complex and use of cytokines in this patient population may result in outcomes considerably different than that of other contexts. The effects of hematopoietic growth factors on pathophysiologic processes relevant to AIDS patients should be considered in weighing the use of these agents in this setting. Among the multiple recognized immune abnormalities associated with HIV infection, dysregulated immunoglobulin expression frequently occurs. Manifest primarily as hypergammaglobulinemia, this phenomena may also result in antibody or immune complex mediated phenomena. One such event is platelet destruction with resultant thrombocytopenia clinically similar to autoimmune idiopathic thrombocytopenia purpura (AITP). This phenomena, which is not associated with advanced immunosuppression or an increased risk of developing AIDS, (Holzman et al) has been hypothesized to be on the basis of immune complex deposition on the platelet surface (Walsh et al) or specific anti-platelet antibodies. (Stricker et al) In addition, immune complex and cell-associated antibodies have been frequently detected on the surfaces of both red cells (McGinniss et al) and neutrophils (Murphy et al, McCance-Katz et al). These have been variably associated with the development of clinical cell count abnormalities. For all cell lineages, the occurrence of cytopenia is inconstantly associated with the presence of antibody or immune complexes on the cell surface. One hypothesis for the discrepancy in the clinical outcome of cell associated antibodies or immune complexes is reticuloendothelial dysfunction also commonly noted in HIV infected patients. (Bender et al, Bender, Quinn et al, Kelton et al) This may result in decreased peripheral clearance of antibody or immune complex coated cells in some patients resulting in the relative preservation of cell counts. The use of hematopoietic growth factors which are known to enhance the function of mature blood cells as well as bone marrow progenitors may have an impact upon this balance. GM-CSF and GCSF may affect opsonization by phagocytic cells. To the extent that cytopenia is caused by clearance of antibody or immune complex coated cells, these growth factors may affect this process in an unpredictable manner.

Abnormal hematopoiesis is thought to play an important role in the development of low blood cell counts in these patients. The development of neutropenia and anemia is associated with progressive immune deficiency. The precise mechanism by which the virus interacts with the hematopoietic system is unclear, however multiple possible mechanisms have been hypothesized. Blood cell progenitor growth and development may be regulated by the interaction of these cells with so-called accessory cells of the marrow environment. Among these, monocyte/macrophages, (Gartner et al, Ho et al) T cells and cells of mesenchymal origin (Clapham et al) have all been documented to be infectable with HIV. Physiologic functions of these cells that may be altered by the presence of HIV including that of cytokine expression. The underexpression of an important trophic factor, the overexpression of an inhibitory factor or the potentially inhibitory effect of overexpression of a trophic factor may all contribute to abnormal regulation of blood cell development. Whether these accessory cells are infected by HIV in vivo and whether infection results in physiologic alterations in cytokonic expression is at this point conjectural. There is, however, in vitro evidence regarding the alteration of interleukin 1-beta (IL-1 beta) and tumor necrosis factor (TNF-alpha) expression in acutely infected monocytoid cells. (Molina et al) The interaction of different cytokines is probably important in determining their effects. Therefore, to the extent that cytokine expression is abnormal and depending upon which particular cytokines are aberrantly expressed, use of exogenous hematopoietic growth factors may have variable consequences in AIDS patients.

Hematopoiesis may also be impaired by the HIV infection of bone cell progenitors. Recent data using MY 10 (CD 34) enriched bone marrow mononuclear cells exposed to high titer virus suggest the infectibility of these early blood elements. (Folks et al) In vivo correlation of this phenomena has not yet been obtained and the consequences of this infection on progenitor cell function are not known. The direct effect of viral infection on progenitor cells may also be influenced by the use of hematopoietic growth factors. In vitro data suggest that viral replication in mononuclear cells may be enhanced by the presence of exogenous factors such as GM-CSF and Interleukin-3 (IL-3), though not by G-CSF. (Koyangi et al) To the extent that hematopoiesis may be affected by the presence of the virus in progenitor cells, the stimulating effect on GM-CSF and IL-3 on viral replication may alter the anticipated effect of GM-CSF administration on blood cell counts.

Coincident complications of HIV infection may also interact with hematopoiesis and the use of growth factors. In particular mycobacterium avium-intracellular and cytomegalovirus are common opportunistic infections in these patients and frequently involve the bone marrow. How exogenous growth factors may interact with these agents or the host response to them is unknown, but may alter the clinical effect of these growth factors. In addition, B cell lymphoma is a common malignancy complicating HIV infection with a high incidence of bone marrow invasion. The use of cytokines in this setting is in the process of being explored.

One of the most clinically important mechanisms of bone marrow suppression in HIV infected patients is that due to therapeutic agents. HIV infected patients tend to be particularly sensitive to the myelo-suppressive effects of agents such as the anti-retroviral azidothymidine (AZT), on trimethoprim/sulfamethoxazole for pneumocystis carinii pneumonia, gancyclovir (DHPG) for cytomegalovirus infection, pyrimethamine/sulfadiazine for central nervous system toxoplasmosis and acyclovir for disseminated herpes simplex or herpes zoster. Myelosuppresion induced by these agents frequently limits their use and indeed, the single approved antiretroviral agent AZT, is commonly limited by neutropenia and anemia. The use of hematopoietic growth factors in the context of these agents is clearly of considerable clinical importance and in may define the therapeutic role of these agents in AIDS patients.

CLINICAL EXPERIENCE:

One of the first clinical trials utilizing recombinant hematopoietic growth factors was conducted in AIDS patients. Neutropenic patients with AIDS or ARC responded to intravenous GM-CSF in a phase I clinical trial with a rapid dose dependent response in leukocyte count. (Groopman et al) Mature and immature neutrophils, eosinophils and monocytes increased within two days of initiating continuous infusion GM-CSF, whereas reticulocyte, lymphocyte and platelet counts were unaltered. Discontinuation of GM-CSF resulted in a decrease of circulating leukocytes to baseline within three to nine days. Short term administration of recombinant human GM-CSF produced by an eukaryotic cell expression system was associated with low grade fever and flu-like symptoms with occasional mild phlebitis and reversible elevations in liver function tests. Bone marrow changes were noted in eleven of fourteen patients with eosinophilia and a shift toward myeloid immaturity occurring commonly.

In addition to the increase in cell numbers, two patients with prior neutrophil functional abnormalities (one in phagocytosis and one in intracellular killing) experienced reversal of the qualitative defect by GM-CSF. (Baldwin et al) Thus leukocyte counts and leukocyte function can be enhanced by the use of GM-CSF in the setting of HIV infection. With this short term use there were no apparent effects on the clinical course of these patients, nor was there a change in the ability to culture HIV from their peripheral mononuclear cells.

A subsequent trial evaluating the use of subcutaneous GM-CSF for a prolonged period of time has been conducted in a similar patient population. (Mitsuyasu et al) A dose dependent response in peak leukocyte count was again seen with no consistent effect on lymphoid, erythroid or platelet elements. Administration of eukaryote-produced recombinant growth factor for greater than six months did not lead to tachyphylaxis and no adverse consequences of prolonged exposure to GM-CSF or the associated eosinophilia were noted. In addition, the serum HIV core antigen (p24) level, a useful indicator of viral activity, showed no consistent alteration over the period of study.

The issue of viral antigen levels in patients receiving GM-CSF has become particularly important in light of recent in vitro evidence of increased viral replication in the presence of GM-CSF and interleukin 3 (IL-3). Preliminary data from a clinical trial utilizing AZT alternating biweekly with GM-CSF indicate increased serum p24 levels during the two weeks of GM-CSF administration. (R. Mitsuya:

personal communication) These levels declined during the period of receiving AZT, suggesting a possible in vivo correlate of viral activation with the use of GM-CSF. These results indicate that GM-CSF should only be used in conjunction with antiretroviral agents. (G-CSF, which does not induce viral replication in vitro, and therefore may have a different effect is currently being evaluated.) The use of GM-CSF in conjunction with the antiretroviral agent AZT is further supported by in vitro data of Perno and colleagues demonstrating an enhanced antiviral effect of AZT in the presence of GM-CSF. (Perno et al) In peripheral blood monocytes the presence of GM-CSF resulted in enhanced intracellular levels of AZT and its active phosphorylated form. The mechanism for this alteration is apparently on the basis of increased cellular uptake of AZT. These biochemical changes result in suppression of viral activity in the presence of GM-CSF at concentrations of AZT ten to one hundredfold lower than when the AZT is present without GM-CSF. This increased intracellular accumulation of AZT is not apparently associated with any increase cytotoxicity and indeed a study by Bhalla has documented decreased levels of phosphorylated AZT in bone marrow mononuclear cells in the presence of GM-CSF. (Bhalla et al) This latter study correlated intracellular levels of AZT with improved bone marrow colony formation in the presence of GM-CSF when contrasted with bone marrow cells grown in the presence of AZT alone.

COMBINATION TRIALS:

Several trials utilizing AZT in combination with GM-CSF are ongoing including one directed by Dr. James D. Levine at New England Deaconess Hospital. In this study, AIDS or ARC patients previously intolerant of AZT therapy due to myelosuppression are given GM-CSF either at the re-initiation of AZT or when neutropenia (absolute neutrophil count (ANC) <1000) has occurred. The recombinant human GM-CSF is derived from a bacterial expression system and is given at 1 mcg/kg/d subcutaneously escalated as necessary to maintain an ANC greater than 1000 cells/mm^3. Preliminary results indicate GM-CSF is able to restore myelopoieses in all patients, however six of seventeen patients did require a dose escalation. Despite restoration of an ANC greater than 1000 cells/mm^3 two bacterial infections have occurred both of which responded to appropriate antibiotic therapy. There have been no opportunistic infections during the period of study and the CD4 counts have not changed (although the starting level is extremely low with a mean of 29 cells/mm^3). The p24 antigen level has not been consistently modulated in the population as a whole. Low grade fever and a flu-like syndrome are common (16/17). Anemia requiring transfusion has developed in 15 of 17 patients and thrombocytopenia (<50,000 cells/mm^3) occurred in 5 of 17 patients. These two phenomena are perhaps related to the unmasking of AZT suppression of these cell lineages, however other etiologies cannot be excluded.

GM-CSF is therefore able to mitigate dose limiting neutropenia in the majority of AIDS/ARC patients who have been previously AZT intolerant. A portion of these patients, however, will develop other cytopenias that may or may not limit the use of AZT. A therapeutic benefit of GM-CSF beyond elevating the neutrophil count cannot be documented by this Phase I/II study.

Further evaluation of GM-CSF in conjunction with other viral therapies in AIDS patients is being conducted in patients with Kaposi's sarcoma combining AZT, interferon alpha and GM-CSF. In this patient population interferon alpha has been demonstrated to have antitumor efficacy in a subset of patients with relatively preserved immune function. (Bhalla) Its benefit has required high doses of interferon (18-36 million units per day) and is frequently associated with treatment limiting flu-like symptoms. Preliminary data has suggested that the benefit of interferon may be extended to a broader spectrum of patients using lower doses of interferon when used in conjunction with AZT. In addition, this combination therapy has been associated with improved immune parameters (CD4 counts) and decreased viral activity (HIV p24 antigen levels). (Krown et al, Deyton et al, Kovacs et al) In vitro, AZT and interferon alpha have a synergistic anti-viral effect when used in combination. Overlapping myelotoxicity of these two agents frequently limits their combined use however and, therefore GM-CSF has been added in a phase I/II clinical trial. In this study, AZT is administered at 1200 mgs/d to which subcutaneously administered interferon alpha at 9 million units/d is added following four weeks of AZT alone. The combination regimen is maintained for twelve weeks during which time GM-CSF is added at any point for an ANC <1000 cells/mm^3. Of sixteen evaluable patients to date, ten have required GM-CSF. Factors on study entry that predict the need for GM-CSF are ANC <2000 cells/mm^3 and CD4 <200 cells/mm^3. The ANC has responded promptly to GM-CSF in all patients. The GM-CSF has in general been well tolerated, however a worsening of the flu-like symptoms of interferon has been noted by two patients. There have been no significant changes in CD4 or p24 antigen levels. Overall 4 of 16 patients have responded and 8 of 16 patients have either had stable or responding disease. Among the nine patients that have received greater than eight weeks of combination of AZT and interferon (the anticipated minimum time for a beneficial anti-tumor effect of interferon) the KS has responded in four of nine and has been stable in four of nine patients. Whether GM-CSF may be associated with an improved response will require larger patient numbers. Though preliminary, these data indicate that GM-CSF is able to mitigate the myelotoxicity of AZT/interferon alpha therapy and is associated with mild, tolerable toxicity. Its ability to improve the therapeutic index of these medications or enhance desired clinical outcomes is as yet undetermined.

SUMMARY

Overall GM-CSF is a well tolerated intervention in patients with HIV associated disease. As in a number of other clinical settings, it is able to improve myelopoiesis and abrogate the myelotoxicity of chemotherapeutic agents. At present, clinical data is insufficient to indicate an ultimate clinical benefit from the use of GM-CSF in terms of opportunistic infection, mortality or quality of life for HIV infected patients. As phase I and phase II trials are completed however comparative clinical trials addressing these issues are anticipated. Hematopoietic growth factors may permit the use of optimal doses of therapeutics and thereby play an adjunctive role in the combination therapies anticipated for the treatment of HIV related disease.

REFERENCES

Baldwin GC, Gasson JC, Quan SG, Fleischman J, Weisbart R, Oette D, Mitsuyasu RT, Golde DW (1988). Granulocyte-macrophage colony-stimulating factor enhances neutrophil function in acquired immunodeficiency syndrome patients. Proc Natl Acad Sci USA 85:2763.

Bender BS, Frank MM, Lawley TJ, Smith WJ, Brickman GM, Quinn TC (1985). Defective reticuloendothelial system Fc-receptor function in patients with acquired immunodeficiency syndrome. J Infect Dis 152(2):409.

Bender BS, Quinn TC, Spivak JL (1987). Homosexual men with thrombocytopenia have impaired reticuloendothelial system Fc receptor-specific clearance. Blood 70:392.

Bhalla K, Bickhofer M, Grant S, Graham G (1989) The effect of recombinant human granulocyte-macrophage colony-stimulating factor (rGM-CSF) on 3'-Azido-3'-deoxythymide AZT)-mediated biochemical and cytotoxic effects on normal human myeloid progenitor cells. Exp Hematol 17:17.

Clapham PR, Weber JN, Whitby D, McIntosh K, Kalgeish AG, Maddon PJ, Deen KC, Sweet RW, Weiss RA (1989). Soluble CD4 blocks the infectivity of diverse strains of HIV and SIV for T-cells and monocytes, but not for brain and muscle cells. Nature 337(26):368.

Deyton L, Kovacs J, Masur H, Metcalf J, Lee D, Salzman N, Baseler M, Bigley J, Lane HC, Gauci AS (1988). Combination trial (Phase I-II) of zidovudine with lymphoblastoid interferon alpha in patients with AIDS and Kaposi's sarcoma. International Conference on AIDS. Stockholm, Sweden abstract 3628.

Folks TM, Kessler SW, Orenstein JM, Justement JS, Jaffe ES, Fauci AS (1988). Infection and replication of HIV-1 in purified progenitor cells of normal human bone marrow. Science 242:919.

Gartner S, Markovis P, Markovitz DM, Kaplan MH, Gallo RC, Popovic M (1986). The role of mononuclear phagocytes in HTLV-III/LAV infection. Science 233(4760):215.

Groopman JE, Mitsuyasu RT, DeLeo MJ, Oette DH, Golde DW (1987). Effect of recominant human granulocyte-macrophage colony-stimulating factor on myelopoiesis in the acquired immunodeficiency syndrome. N Engl J Med 317(10):593.

Ho DD, Rota TR, Hirsch MS (1986). Infection of monocyte/macrophages by human T-lymphotropic virus type III. J Clin Invest 77(5):1712.

Holzman RS, Walsh CM, Karpatkin S (1987). Risk for the acquired immunodeficiency syndrome among thrombocytopenic and non-thrombocytopenic homosexual men seropositive for the human immunodeficiency virus. Ann Intern Med 106:383.

Kelton JG, Carter CF, Rodger C, et al (1984). The relationship among platelet-assoicated IgG, platelet lifespan, and reticuloendothelial cell function. Blood 63:1434.

Kovacs JA, Deyton L, Davey R, et al (1989). Combined zidovudine and interferon-*a* therapy in patients with Kaposi's sarcoma and the acquired immunodeficiency syndrome (AIDS). Annals of Internal Medicine; 111:280-287.

Koyangi Y, O'Brian WA, Zhao JW, et al (1988). Cytokines alter production of HIV-1 from primary mononuclear phagocytes. Science 241:1673.

Krown S, Bundow D, Gansbacher B, Tong W, et al (1988). Interferon-*a* plus zidovudine: A phase I trial in aids-associated Kaposi's sarcoma (KS). IV International Conference on AIDS. Stockholm, Sweden, abstract 3627.

McCance-Katz EF, Hoecker JL, Vitale NB (1987). Severe neutropenia-associated with anti-neutrophil antibody in a patient with acquired immunodeficiency syndrome-related complex. Pediatr Infect Dise J 6(4):417.

McGinniss MH, Macher AM, Rook AH, Alter HJ (1986). Red cell auto-antibodies in patients with acquired immune deficiency syndrome. Transfusion 26(5):405.

Mitsuyasu RT, DeLeo MJ, Miles S, Levine J, Oette D, Golde D, Groopman JE (1988). Chronic dose subcutaneous administration of recombinant GM-CSF in patients with HIV-related leukopenia. IV International Congress on AIDS, Stockholm, Sweden (abstr).

Molina JM, Scadden DT, Byrn RA, Dinarello CA, Groopman JE (1989). Production of tumor necrosis factor @ and interleukin 1*B* by monocytic cells infected with human immunodeficiency virus. J Clin Invest 84:733-737.

Murphy MF, Metcalfe P, Walters AH, Carne CA, Weller IV, Linch DC, Smith A (1987). Incidence and mechanism of neutropenia and thrombocytopenia in patients with human immunodeficiency virus infection. Br J Haematol 66(3):337.

Perno CF, Yarchoan R, Cooney DA, Hartman N, Webb DSA, Hao Z, Mitsuya H, Johns DG, Broder S (1989). Replication of human immunodeficiency in monocytes. J Exp Med 169:933.

Stricker RB, Abrams DI, Corash L, Shuman MA (1985). Target platelet antigen in homosexual men with immune thrombocytopenia. N Engl J Med 313(22):1375.

Walsh CM, Nardi MA, Karpatkin S (1984). On the mechanism of thrombocytopenic purpura in sexually active homosexual men. N Engl J Med 311(10):635.

Index

Acanthosis nigricans
  anti-transferrin receptors in, 92
Accessory cells
  growth factors and, 4–5
Acetyltransferase
  chloramphenicol (CAT), 32–33
Acute myeloblastic leukemia (AML), 54, 156
Additive effects
  of cross-lineage stimulation, 2–3
Adventitious translocation, 22
Agranulocytosis, 143–149
AIDS. *See* Anemia, AIDS
AITP. *See* Autoimmune idiopathic thrombocytopenia purpura
Alcoholism
  GM-CSF therapy, 28
Allergic rhinitis
  IgG fraction in, 92
Amino acid
  in human epo, 20
AML. *See* Acute myeloblastic leukemia
Amniotic fluid
  M-CSF levels, 45
Anemia
  AIDS
    erythropoietin therapy, 113–119
    GM-CSF therapy, 28, 163–172
    granulocyte counts in, 124–125
    HIV infection, 114–115, 165
    mechanisms, 114–115
  aplastic, 28, 143–149
  from combination drug trials, 170
  epo therapy, 21
  hemolytic, 115
Antibiotics
  in AIDS anemia, 114–115
Antigens, viral
  in GM-CSF, 168–169
Anti-transferrin receptors, 92–93
Aplastic anemia, 28, 143–149
Arteriosclerosis
  from erythropoietin therapy, 110
Asparagine residues, 20
Asthma
  IgG fraction in, 92
AT-rich region
  of GM-CSF, 32
Autoimmune idiopathic thrombocytopenia purpura (AITP), 169
Autologous marrow cells
  IgG fraction, effect, 88
  megakaryocytic colony formation, effects, 87
Autologous transfusion
  hematocrit levels, 110
  methods, 106–108
  potential problems, 105–106
  red cell volume, 109–110
  units collected, 108–109
Azidothymidine (AZT)
  in AIDS anemia, 114–115
  combined with GM-CSF, 169–172
  myelo-suppressive effects, 167

B12 levels
  in AIDS anemia, 115
B cell lymphoma
  interacting with hematopoiesis, 166

Biological activities
  granulocyte-macrophage, 28–29
  interleukin-7, 68–71
  macrophage, 51–52
Blood pressure
  in erythropoietin therapy, 110
B lymphocyte pathways
  interleukins defined as, 2
Body fluids, 43–45
Bone cell progenitor
  HIV infection, 166
Bone marrow, cellularity
  failure
    in AIDS anemia, 114–115
    GM-CSF therapy, 28
  in hyperplasia, 146
  transplantation, 121–126
Burns
  GM-CSF therapy, 28
  M-CSF levels, 45
Burst-forming units, 131, 154–155

CAT. *See* Chloramphenicol acetyltransferase
Cells
  activation, 3, 5–6, 52–54
  in AIDS, 164
  antibodies associated with, 164
  in CSF secretion, 139
  See also specific cells
Central system toxoplasmosis
  pyrimethamine/sulfadiazine therapy, 167
Cerebrospinal fluid
  M-CSF levels, 45
Chemotaxis, 156
Chemotherapy
  CSF potential, 122–126
  GM-CSF therapy, 28
Chloramphenicol acetyltransferase (CAT), 32–33
Chromosome 5
  GM-CSF on, 32–36
  M-CSF on, 50
Circulating epo, 22–23
Clinical trials
  combination
  AZT and GM-CSF, 169–172
  M-CSF, 6–7, 56
Cloning
  of human epo, 21
Clonogenic cells, 131
Colony forming units
  GEMM, 130
  spleen, 129–130
Colony stimulating factors (CSF)
  characteristics, 121–122
  in chemotherapy, 122–126
  cross-lineage, 2–3
  gene regulation by, 135–136
  granulocyte (G-CSF)
    cell activation, 5–6
    clinical trials, 6–7
    defined, 1
    differentiative effects, 154–158
    macrophage activities, 3
    monocyte activities, 3
    multilineage action, 2
    in myelodysplastic syndromes, 151–158
    production, 4–5
    at progenitor/stem cell level, 3
    proliferative effects, 154–158
  granulocyte-macrophage (GM-CSF)
    in AIDS, 28, 163–172
    antigen viral levels, 168–169
    AZT combined with, 169–172
    biochemical studies, 34
    biological activities, 28–29
    in bone marrow transplantation, 121–126
    cell proliferation from, 131–132
    cells of, 5–6, 30–31
    in chemotherapy, 123–124
    chromosome 5 in, 32–36
    clinical trials, 6–7
    clinical uses, 28–29
    cytokines affecting, 79–80
    defined, 1, 24–25
    differentiative effects, 154–158
    hematopoietic role, 28–31
    IgG fraction effects, 88
    interleukin-1 effects, 35–36
    in Kaposi's sarcoma, 170–171
    multilineage action, 2
    in oxidative bursts, 125
    in phagocytosis, 125
    production, 4–5, 50–51
    proliferative effects, 154–158

regulation of expression, 24–37
sequences controlling, 32–36
serum blocking actions, 89
subcutaneous, 168
toxicity, 148
macrophage (M-CSF)
animal studies, 54–56
biological activities, 51–52
in body fluids, 43–45
cell activation, 3, 5–6, 52–54
clinical trials, 6–7, 56
evolution, 49–50
genetic location, 49–50
as growth factor, 51–52
human mRNA, 48
leukemogenesis and, 54
maintenance function, 52
preclinical studies, 54–56
in pregnancy, 45
production, 4–5
stimulatory effects, 54–56
structure, 45–48
toxicity, 56
megakaryocyte (MK-CSF)
in AIDS anemia, 115
identification, 78
maturation, 85–93
regulation, 85–86
molecular weights, 78–79
neutrophilic stimulation, 131–133
production, 129–139
sources, 133–139
Coomb's test
in AIDS anemia, 115
Cross-lineage stimulation, 2–3
Cryptococcus neoformans, 125
CSF-1. *See* Colony stimulating factors, macrophage
C-terminal deletion, 48
Cyclical hematopoiesis, 91
Cyclical thrombocytopenia, 91
Cyclic amegakaryocytic thrombocytopenia, 87–93
Cyclic neutropenia, 91
Cytogenetic abnormalities, 158
Cytomegalovirus
gancyclovir therapy, 167
interacting with hematopoiesis, 166
Cytokines
in B cell lymphoma, 166
in megakaryocyte inhibition, 84
of MK-CSF, 73–78
producing CSFs, 138
Cytopenias
in HIV infection, 163–172
refractory, 152

Diabetes
GM-CSF therapy, 28
Disulfide bonds, 20
DNase I footprinting, 34
DNA sequences, 21
cDNA coding
of IL7, 67–78
Dysplasia, myeloid
in AIDS anemia, 115
Dyspnea, 147
Dysregulated immunoglobulin expression, 169

Endotoxin
CSF regulation by, 134
in detecting growth factors, 4
Endothelial cells
expressing GM-CSF, 30–31
Enriched immature myeloid cell populations (EIMCP), 154
Eosinophilic hyperplasia, 146–148
Erythroid pathway, 3
Erythropoietin
in AIDS anemia, 113–119
AZT dosage, 118–119
cloning, 21
disulfide bonds, 20
DNA sequences, 21
interleukins, interactions with, 3
megakaryocytopoiesis
effects of, 81–83
molecular mechanisms, 22
oligosaccharides of, 20–21
origins, 21–22
potency, 19–20
properties, 20
recombinant human (rHuEPO)
platelets vs., 118
detection, 110
efficacy, 111

side effects, 118–119
structure, 107–108
secretion, 22–23
transformed cells, 22
translocation, 22

Fatigue, 147
Fetal liver
epo from, 21
Fibroblasts
expressing GM-CSF, 30–31
Fisher's exact test
for erythropoietin, 108
Footprinting
DNase I, 34

Gancyclovir
in cytomegalovirus, 167
G-CSF. *See* Colony stimulating factor, granulocyte
Gel retardation, 22
Gene regulation, 135–136
Genetic location
of M-CSF, 49–50
GM-CSF. *See* Colony stimulating factor, granulocyte-macrophage
Granulocyte colony stimulating factor. *See* Colony stimulating factor, granulocyte
Granulocyte-macrophage colony stimulating factor. *See* Colony stimulating factor, granulocyte-macrophage
Granulocytic hyperplasia, 146–148
Growth factors
accessory cells, effect on, 4–5
M-CSF-induced, 51–52
model, 6–7
production, 4–5
therapy of, in aplastic anemia, 148–149

Hematocrit levels, 110
Hematopoiesis
in AIDS, 165
biology, 1–18
defective proliferation, 154
GM-CSF in, 28–31
interleukin-7, 71
model, 4–6
stromal cells in, 5–6
Hemolytic anemia, 115
Hemorrhage, 147
Hepatitis
non-A non-B, 147
Hepatoma cell line, 22
HIV-related anemia. *See* Anemia, AIDS
Humoral regulation
of megakaryocytopoiesis, 75–77
Hybridization. *See In situ* hybridization
Hypergammaglobulinemia, 169
Hyperplasia
granulocytic, 146–148
Hypoxic stress, 21–22

IgG fraction
effects, 88–93
IL. *See* Interleukin
Immune complex antibodies
in AIDS, 164
Immunoglobulin expression
dysregulated, 169
Infections
intraabdominal, 147
M-CSF levels, 45
Inhibitors
megakaryocyte, 83–84
In situ hybridization
epo levels, 22
M-CSF levels, 45
Interferon
CSF regulation by, 134
in detecting growth factors, 4
Interferon-alpha
in Kaposi's sarcoma, 170–171
Interleukin-1 (IL-1)
CSF regulation by, 134
in detecting growth factors, 4
effects on GM-CSF messenger, 35–36
expressing GM-CSF, 30–31
Interleukin 1–beta
in immune deficiency, 165
Interleukin-3 (IL-3)
cell proliferation from, 131–132
cytokines affecting, 79–80
defined, 1
multilineage action, 2
production, 5
Interleukin-6
cell production, 5–6
CSF regulation by, 134
MK-CSA in, 80–81
Interleukin-7

in vitro biology, 68–70
in vivo biology, 70–71
isolation, 66–67
molecular characterization, 67–68
Intraabdominal infection, 147
Iron deficiency
anti-transferrin receptors in, 92

Jaundice, 147
Jurkat T-cells, 33

Kaposi's sarcoma
from combination drug trials, 170–171
Kidney
epo from, 21–22

Lectine
in detecting growth factors, 4
Leukemia
acute myeloblastic (AML), 54, 156
Leukemogenesis
M-CSF and, 54
Leukocytes
migration, 124–125
in neutrophil abnormalities, 168
Leukocytosis, 147, 148
Lymphoid pathways, 2
Lymphoproliferative disorders
GM-CSF therapy, 28

Macrophage colony stimulating factor. *See* Colony stimulating factor, macrophage
M-CSF. *See* Colony stimulating factor, macrophage
Megakaryocytopoiesis
erythropoietin effects, 81–83
humoral regulation, 75–77
inhibitors, 83–84
Methionine
in human epo, 20
Mice
amino acid residues, 20
M-CSF levels, 45
MK-CSF. *See* Colony stimulating factor, megakaryocyte
MLA 144 cells, 34
Monkey
amino acid residues, 20
Monocyte(s)
activities, 3
M-CSF, 51
Multi-CSF. *See* Interleukin-3
Multilineage action, 2
Myalgia, 147
Myasthenia gravis
IgG fraction in, 92
Mycobacterium avium-intracellulare
in AIDS anemia, 114
interacting with hematopoiesis, 166
Myeloblastic leukemia
acute (AML), 54, 156
Myelodysplastic syndromes, 151–158
Myeloid dysplasia
in AIDS anemia, 115
Myeloid effector cells, 28
Myeloid pathways, 2
Myocardial infarction
from erythropoietin therapy, 110

Neutropenia
cyclic, 91
GM-CSF therapy, 28
in immune deficiency, 165
Neutrophils
abnormally functioning, 168
stimulation, 131–133
Non-A non-B hepatitis, 147
Non-hematopoietic cells, 139

Oligosaccharides, 20–21
Oxidative bursts, 125

Pericarditis, 147
Peripheral artery thrombosis
from erythropoietin therapy, 110
Phagocytosis, 125, 156
Plasmacytosis
in AIDS anemia, 115
Pneumocystis carinii pneumonia
trimethoprim/sulfadiazine therapy, 167
Polypeptide structure
epo, 21
M-CSF, 48
Pregnancy
M-CSF levels, 45
Promoter constructs, 33–34
Proteins
M-CSF, 45–48
Pulmonary infiltrates, 147, 148
Pyrimethamine/sulfadiazine
in central system toxoplasmosis, 167

Radioimmunoassay
in erythropoietin therapy, 110
Radiotherapy
GM-CSF therapy, 28
Recombinant epo. *See* Erythropoietin, recombinant human
Red blood cells
in AIDS anemia, 115
erythropoietin therapy, 109–110
Refractory cytopenias, 152
Regulation
in megakaryocytopoiesis
humoral, 75–77
in megakaryocyte maturation, 85–86
Residues
asparagine, 20
Reticuloendothelial function
in platelet destruction, 92
rHuEPO. *See* Erythropoietin, recombinant human
RNA
for M-CSF, 48

Sarcoma, Kaposi's from combination drug trials, 170–171
Secretion
epo, 22–23
Serum M-CSF levels, 45
Sialic acid terminal oligosaccharides, 20–21
Spleen colony forming units, 129–130
Stem cells, 3
Stress, hypoxic, 21–22
Stromal cells, 5–6
isolation, 66–67
Subcutaneous GM-CSF, 168
Synergistic effects
of cross-lineage stimulation, 2–3

Target cells, 3
T cells
GM-CSF and, 32–33, 134, 136
pathways for, 2
T-gamma syndrome, 145
Thrombocytopenia
in AIDS anemia, 115, 169
from combination drug trials, 170
cyclic amegakaryocytic, 87–93
rhGM-CSF induced, 147
Thrombopoiesis
clinical disorders, 87–93
in megakaryocyte maturation, 85–86
Thrombosis, peripheral artery
from erythropoietin therapy, 110
Tissues
GM-CSF expressing 30–31
TNF
effects on GM-CSF messenger, 35–36
Toxicity
aplastic anemia, 147
M-CSF, 56
Toxoplasmosis, central system
pyrimethamine/sulfadiazine, 167
TPA
expressing GM-CSF, 30–31
Transfusion, autologous. *See* Autologous transfusion
Transcripts
M-CSF, 45–48
Transformed cells, 22
Transplantation
bone marrow, 121–126
Trimethoprim/sulfamethoxazole
myelo-suppressive effects, 167
Tuberculosis
in AIDS anemia, 114
Tumor(s)
GM-CSF therapy, 28
Tumor necrosis factor
in detecting growth factors, 4
expressing GM-CSF, 30–31
Tumor necrosis factor-alpha
in immune deficiency, 165

Urinary epo. *See* Epo, urinary

Viral antigens levels in GM-CSF, 168–169

WI-38 cell line, 34–35
Wilcoxson midranks test
for erythropoietin, 108